A Right to Health

Book Thirty-seven, Louann Atkins Temple Women & Culture Series

A Right to Health

Medicine, Marginality, and
Health Care Reform
in Northeastern Brazil

JESSICA SCOTT JEROME

University of Texas Press ◆ *Austin*

The Louann Atkins Temple Women & Culture Series is supported by Allison, Doug, Taylor, and Andy Bacon; Margaret, Lawrence, Will, John, and Annie Temple; Larry Temple; the Temple-Inland Foundation; and the National Endowment for the Humanities.

First edition, 2015
First paperback printing, 2016

Requests for permission to reproduce material from this work should be sent to:
    Permissions
    University of Texas Press
    P.O. Box 7819
    Austin, TX 78713-7819
    http://utpress.utexas.edu/index.php/rp-form

♾ The paper used in this book meets the minimum requirements of ANSI/NISO Z39.48-1992 (R1997) (Permanence of Paper).

Library of Congress Cataloging-in-Publication Data

Jerome, Jessica Scott, author.
    A right to health : medicine, marginality, and health care reform in northeastern Brazil / by Jessica S. Jerome. — First edition.
        p. ; cm. — (Louann Atkins Temple women & culture series ; book 37)
    Includes bibliographical references and index.
    ISBN 978-0-292-76662-4 (cloth : alk. paper)
    ISBN 978-0-292-76663-1 (library e-book)
    ISBN 978-0-292-76664-8 (non-library e-book)
    I. Title.   II. Series: Louann Atkins Temple women & culture series ; bk. 37.
    [DNLM: 1. Health Care Reform—history—Brazil.   2. Delivery of Health Care—Brazil.   3. Health Policy—history—Brazil.   4. Universal Coverage—Brazil.   WA 541 DB8]
    RA418.3.B6
    362.10981—dc23
                                                                                                2014026812
    ISBN 978-1-4773-1131-8, paperback

doi:10.7560/766624

For my parents, Jon and Julie Jerome

Contents

Acknowledgments

I owe the completion of this book to the many individuals who saw me through it. My deepest gratitude is extended to each of them.

In Brazil my debts are numerous and difficult to encompass within these brief words. Prior to conducting fieldwork, I spent two summers completing language training in Rio de Janeiro and São Paulo. In both of these cities I had the good fortune of meeting people who encouraged my research interests and shared with me the beauty of their country. I thank in particular Gilda and Emmanuel Santos, Christina Rizzi, and Suzana Sumoraes. I also want to thank Antônio José Lapa, who kindly showed me around his laboratory in São Paulo and patiently answered my many ill-formed questions.

During my first visit to Fortaleza I had the great luck to meet Francisco Abreu Matos and Adalberto Barreto. Dr. Abreu Matos, a natural-products chemist at the Universidade Federal do Ceará, was a charming and genteel man whose quiet discipline remains an inspiration. His great patience in answering my questions and his gentle encouragement of my research in Ceará sustained me throughout my first period of fieldwork. Adalberto Barreto, a professor of social medicine and a psychiatrist, introduced me to Pirambu and ensured that I could live there while I was conducting fieldwork. I thank him for trusting a relative stranger to be a guest in the community on whose behalf he worked tirelessly and for ferrying countless letters back and forth between his home, which I initially used as an address to receive mail, and my own in Pirambu. I benefited a great deal from his unobtrusive support and learned much from his sincere and energetic engagement with the residents of Pirambu.

I also want to thank Professor Luiz A. de Castro Santos, a historian at the Universidade Estadual do Rio de Janeiro. As soon as I found my way to his careful and insightful studies of public health in Brazil, Professor Castro Santos became a generous and patient interlocutor. His work continues to shape my thought on the topics in this book.

From my first days in Pirambu I was embraced by Irene Marquez dos Santos and her daughter, Joelma Brandão. It was their presence that enabled me to make it through the first few difficult months of fieldwork. I thank also the entire Brandão family, Maria José, her sons Wellington and Neves, and Neves's wife, Nézia. During my first period of fieldwork I spent many twilight hours with Neves's and Nézia's daughters, Vanessa, Andressa, and Alessandra, whom I thank for showering me with laughter and light. Daví and Fabiana extended their friendship and were endlessly curious about the worlds we shared as well as those we did not. I deeply admire their conviction, and they are just two examples of the extraordinary intellects and spirits that survive in Pirambu. Thanks are also due to Cezário, who brought me my first pair of flip-flops and helped me to find my feet in the favela.

Finally, I thank Francinete Mota, Gliciane Lima do Nascimento, Glícia Lima do Nascimento, Alindaiza Barros, Jucilene Mota Vaz, and Lúcia Santos for their friendship. Time spent in the company of these women in Pirambu and in parts of Ceará I would not have otherwise seen are among the memories I treasure most. It was wholly on the strength of all these relationships that this research became worth undertaking.

This book was written over many years and has had many different interlocutors, each of whom has been important to the development of my ideas and research. At the University of Chicago, where I completed the dissertation upon which the early research for this book was based, I thank my adviser, Manuela Carneiro da Cunha. She arranged introductions and connections in Brazil without which I could not have begun the project. I thank her for her encouragement throughout the many different stages of my research. I also thank members of my thesis committee, John Kelly, Terrence Turner, and Elizabeth Povinelli, all extraordinary teachers who revealed how to turn the end of an inquiry into a beginning and shaped my commitment to anthropology.

Following the completion of my graduate work, I was a fellow at the MacLean Center for Clinical Medical Ethics under the direction of Mark Siegler. There I was fortunate to be connected to Stacy Tessler Lindau, an obstetrician and medical researcher who opened up another world of scholarship to me and helped me to see anthropology anew.

More recently she was generous enough to provide an office for me as I revised the manuscript for publication. I thank Mark and Stacy for welcoming me into their community and for demonstrating other ways to think about the question of human being.

And finally, I thank Laura Nader for introducing me to the practice of anthropology as an undergraduate and for demonstrating its enormous potential as a human endeavor and its fundamental humanity. Though each of these mentors practices a different kind of social science, they all share a commitment to social justice and a belief in the transformative capacity of scholarship that continues to inspire my work. I would also like to gratefully acknowledge the financial support received for various stages of this research, including that from the Rio Branco Institute and the National Science Foundation.

For taking two chances on this manuscript I am deeply grateful to the support and encouragement of Theresa J. May at the University of Texas Press. I also thank Leslie Tingle for ushering the book into print. The manuscript benefited enormously from the detailed reports of two anonymous readers.

I have also benefited enormously from the support and engagement of a number of friends. For visits home and extended discussions about themes that pervade this book I thank Sara O'Connor Johnson and Shree Ram. For their friendship and patient help in seeing me through graduate school I thank Emiliano Corral, Breena Holland, Kathleen Lowrey, and Debra McDougall. The Environmental Studies Workshop, in its early incarnations and when I returned from the field, provided a warm and lively space to present new work and to debate a wide range of theoretical concerns and issues. When I embarked on fieldwork there were many times when anthropology seemed like a futile and lonely endeavor; I am immensely grateful to Kathleen Lowrey for her correspondence during this time and since then. Her piercing wit and intellect continue to remind me of the joys of seeing the world from an anthropological point of view.

I began teaching in northern New Mexico at St. John's College, and I feel only great fortune at having been a part of that academic community. Despite the absence of anthropology in its curricula, I was encouraged to think deeply about many of the themes that haunt this work. For countless hours of deep friendship, laughter, and community I thank Keri Ames, Jan Arsenault, Christine Chen, Stephan Houser, Andy Kingston, Laurence Nee (1970–2013), and Gregory Schneider.

Elsa Davidson and Paul Kockelman are two friends from childhood who are practicing anthropologists. Though committed to different modes of inquiry, their scholarship and wise counsel have reminded me over the years of what this field can be at its very best.

I am so very grateful as well to the families that have seen this project through from start to finish. I thank the Holz family, Frank, Julia, Ben, and Rachel, for support and encouragement at times when very little was due, for the countless hours of child care they provided while I worked to finish parts of the manuscript, and for all the happy diversions along the way. I want to thank Julia Holz in particular for organizing a series of talks during the summer of 2010 in Manila that helped me to formulate my ideas and think more carefully about the connections between health care and human rights.

My mother and father, who in addition to taking care of grandchildren have patiently read through every draft of these chapters and offered thoughtful, rigorous, and engaging criticisms. I could not have undertaken a project of this magnitude without their support.

Finally, I thank Daniel Holz for encouraging me from the very beginning to the very end of this work. His unstinting curiosity about our world animates every aspect of this book. Samuel and Ishmael, thank you for your presence in this world, and with your father, I thank you for being in it all together.

A Right to Health

Introduction

In 1988 Brazil adopted a new constitution that defined health care as a right of all citizens and the responsibility of the state. It further established a new health care system, the Sistema Único de Saúde (SUS, Unified Health Care System), which dramatically transformed all aspects of the way health care was practiced, from the way funding was allocated to the categories of citizens to whom medical care was extended to the very way that health itself was imagined.

Brazil's transformation of its health care system was a profoundly radical step, not just in the context of the country's emergence from twenty years of military dictatorship but also in a global context of widespread reevaluation of the welfare state leading to a shift to privatized models of health care throughout Latin America and the world.[1] As such, Brazil's reforms have been the subject of extensive analysis and political debate, and its consequences have been measured and assessed.[2] What has received less attention are the insights that health care reform offers into more general questions about the nature of universal rights, social belonging, and citizenship in the everyday lives of individuals, families, and communities.

This book is an ethnography of health care reform in the state of Ceará, a midsize state in Northeast Brazil. In it I investigate the meanings and possibilities of new ideologies and practices of health care. I focus on a population for whom the reforms were intended to matter most: the residents of Brazil's peripheral communities,[3] in this case, on the margins of Fortaleza, Ceará's capital city. The reforms associated with the SUS have increased access to medical care and technologies for low-income residents in Fortaleza and elsewhere in Brazil (Victora 2011); they have promoted new models of citizen participation in the formulation of health care policy (Coelho 2007, Cornwall 2007). Yet these reforms emerged in the context of neoliberal economic policies that encouraged the ongoing privatization of health care and consequently weakened the country's already fragile political culture of civil rights (Caldeira and Holston 1999, Holston 2008, Scheper-Hughes 2006).[4] At the local level, the SUS reforms have become entangled with residents' visions of community activism and their future-oriented aspirations, both of which have grown out of experiences of exclusion from political and economic structures.

The complex relationship between a formal right to health and the ways this right is experienced within a community became evident early on in my fieldwork. Some of these complexities are encapsulated in the following story. Several months after arriving in Pirambu, the community where I lived and conducted most of my fieldwork, an older man named Benito Antonelli came to stay with my next-door neighbor Elizabete. Benito was from Crato, a small town in the far south of the state of Ceará. Elizabete was his second cousin. Some time prior to Benito's arrival, a young schoolteacher in Crato who knew Benito wrote to Elizabete on his behalf and asked if he might stay with her in Pirambu for a short time while he was seeking medical treatment in Fortaleza. The city, she wrote, would have sophisticated medical care accessible even to "pessoas bem pobres" (very poor people) like Benito. Elizabete agreed to host him, and Benito arrived shortly thereafter.

When Benito arrived he was already in poor health. He had what he said was an ear infection and had waited almost two months at home in Crato before deciding to do anything about it. The day after his arrival, Elizabete took him to the nearest primary care clinic, where a nurse's assistant carefully washed his ear, covered it with pads of gauze and adhesive tape, and recommended aspirin for the pain. That was the first medical attention his ear had received. He was instructed to go to a local medical clinic to be seen by a doctor.

Several days later Elizabete and I accompanied Benito to the clinic a short bus ride away from the neighborhood. We took a number from the receptionist and sat in the hot, open-air waiting room for most of the morning. While we waited, Elizabete marveled at the clinic, which apparently had been built only five years earlier. She explained, "When I first arrived in Fortaleza [in 1961] we were just starting to get [public] health clinics in the favela. We protested a lot back then because before that there was nothing. You might as well have been in the *interior*."[5] As I was to learn in the course of our many subsequent conversations, she was an active participant in Pirambu's social movements during the early 1960s; she was also one of the few residents I met who explicitly linked the construction of the new health clinic to the Sistema Único de Saúde.

By the time Benito's number was called that morning, the doctor had left for the day, and we were instructed to return to the clinic the next day. It took several more visits before Benito was finally seen, by which point he was told that his case looked "very serious and complicated." He would need to see a specialist and was given a referral to a doctor at one of the city's main hospitals. The clinic's doctor gave Benito a prescription for a pain reliever that was supposed to be available for free in the clinic's pharmacy. Elizabete didn't bother to stop, however, as she assured me the pharmacy's shelves were almost always empty.

That evening Elizabete narrated the day's events to her twenty-two-year-old daughter, Fabiana. She asked Fabiana to call her boyfriend, who worked as a driver for a family she described as "gente boa" (good people); the man was an administrator at the hospital to which Benito had been referred. "Maybe he'd find a way to get Benito in a little earlier," Elizabete reasoned. "He can't wait here in Fortaleza for too long, and his ear is getting worse." The call was apparently made in the next several days and an appointment set for Benito to go to the hospital the following week. I couldn't accompany him on that visit, but Elizabete said later that the doctor suspected a cancerous tumor and wanted to do blood tests and an MRI. More appointments were made for the next few weeks, but Benito would have to wait two months for the MRI exam.

One evening Fabiana began complaining to me about the public health system through which Benito was getting care. "It's so typical," she said, "all this waiting and the incompetent doctors. Why can't they just tell him what's wrong?" She continued, "Look, it [his medical care] has *cara de favela*." This phrase, literally "face of a favela," was one I was to hear often during repeated field visits to Pirambu to describe anything that was particularly ineffectual or dilapidated.

In the fifth week of his visit Benito turned visibly worse, becoming unable to swallow anything and complaining of severe pain. Although he had not yet completed any of the medical tests advised by the doctor he'd seen at the hospital, he decided he would nonetheless return to Crato. Elizabete asked him if he was sure, if he didn't want to try to get an earlier appointment for any of the tests; perhaps they could find a way. But he demurred, and the next night he left by bus for Crato.

When I discussed Benito's case sometime later with a doctor who worked in Pirambu, he only shrugged and said, "All the people here want is drugs. They think that is what medical care is. This is why our work is so hard. We're trying to provide something else—preventive medicine. We try to teach people how to take care of their bodies so they won't need so many drugs in the long run."

Reflecting on this sequence of events, I was initially surprised by how much medical care an impoverished man like Benito received during his relatively short stay in Fortaleza, a city he had never before visited. On the other hand, I had to agree with Fabiana that in the end, relatively little was accomplished. Benito had been seen by several doctors but never given a diagnosis; his tests remained incomplete, including blood tests and an expensive MRI exam; and he left without any medication or hope for a cure. Perhaps most surprisingly, Benito himself seemed content when he left the favela. He defined his visit as a success and remarked pointedly on the quantity and quality of resources he had received while in Fortaleza.

I highlight this story because it puts into relief that health care is never only about finding a cure, negotiating treatment, or allocating resources. It is also a site at which social class, generational tension, aspiration, and citizenship are expressed and reproduced. In the months following Benito's departure I continued to return to a series of questions: How had Benito, living in the rural backland of a relatively poor Northeastern state, come to imagine Fortaleza as a place that would have accessible medical care? Why was Fabiana's perspective on the public health care system so different from that of her mother? And what was entailed in the doctor's vision of preventive medicine, and how was it connected to the rights discourse that I was beginning to observe in selected venues in Fortaleza?

Each of these questions could only be answered when I considered the daily structuring of class, gender, and generation in the favela as well as the historical origins of putatively new concepts such as democracy and citizenship. Participant observation and extended interviews over many years in the same field site allowed me to observe social patterns that illuminated the broad relationship between health and citizenry. By grounding my research in one particular community, I hope to contribute an ethnographic dimension to discussions of health care reform that have largely focused on quantitative assessments of outcomes and expenditures and consistently have framed Brazil's neoliberal economic policies as independent of or irrelevant to the constitutional claim for health care rights. It is an examination of precisely the other, ethnographic themes that I argue will help us to understand if and to what extent a "right to health" is rooted in peripheral residents' ideas and practices of health care.

Human Rights as Cultural Practice

One way of thinking about political rights, civil rights (sometimes referred to as social rights), or even more broadly human rights is as a cultural practice that organizes an individual's relationship to the collective life of which she or he is a part (Preis 1996). Viewing rights as a form of practice shifts attention away from deliberation over the moral worth of abstract models and toward an understanding of how rights are put to work in people's everyday lives. Like all cultural practices, rights find their meaning in situated contexts that an ethnographer must elucidate in order to understand how they enter into the life-worlds of individuals and social groups.

As I discuss in chapter 2 of this book, the Brazilian welfare state that emerged under President Getúlio Vargas during the 1930s organized its benefits scheme in terms that suggested an ethos of mutual responsibility across social classes and generations. One of the basic premises underlying this form of social protection was that the risks inherent in living and working in a market-based society could and should be reapportioned from those who were protected from risk and economic uncertainty to those who were less fortunate and unable to bear those risks alone (S. Brooks 2008). In practice this reapportionment was restricted to private-sector workers who through their contributions of labor and taxes were repaid by assistance from the state in the form of medical care, unemployment wages, and retirement funds (Holston 2008).

During the 1930s and 1940s Pirambu was just emerging as a community, and few of its residents were members of the classes of laborers who benefited from the social protection schemes conceived by President Vargas. If we look at newspaper coverage of that time, however, journalists report that starting in the early 1940s residents began to lobby for a broad spectrum of civil rights, including the right to ownership of the land on which they were living, reliable transportation, running water, electricity, and access to basic health services.

This activity—public demonstrations for services from a city that had yet to recognize personhood, let alone citizenship—is a form of cultural practice that uses public appearance to draw attention to the contradictions in the arrangements that exclude them. Both Hannah

Arendt in her classic 1951 work, *The Origins of Totalitarianism*, and James Holston in his 2008 ethnography of insurgent citizenship in urban Brazil have referred to this practice as advocating for the "right to have rights." Although not a formal model of "rights," it is world-changing nonetheless: by acting as if they had the rights that they lacked, residents of Pirambu managed to actualize aspects of civil equality to which they aspired, such as access to legal housing, cleaner water, public transportation, and medical clinics. Holston summarizes this activity during a later period, the 1970s, in the city of Sao Paulo: "In this performance they produced a transformation in the understanding of Brazilian citizenship itself of great social consequence, from a distribution of privilege to particular categories of citizens to a distribution of the right to rights for all citizens" (241).

More than a century after the initiation of the welfare state and in part as a response to the decades-long swell of activism among the urban poor, the Brazilian government partially amended the practice of selective reapportionment of worker benefits by turning one category of benefits, health care, into a right of citizenship rather than of employment. Ideally this amendment affirmed the principle that with regard to health, society ought to provide security to all members of the Brazilian nation-state regardless of their ability to contribute remunerative labor to the state. But in practice Pirambu's older residents rarely sought health care on these terms, and younger, more affluent residents of the community tended to eschew the idea of a collective good altogether in favor of consuming the medical care of their choice. In writing an ethnography of health care reform and of the rights it is purported to enact, I have drawn attention throughout to the disjuncture in the ideal and the practice of health care rights in Pirambu and to the historical origins of both abstract concept and social practice.

From Patronage to Neoliberalism, Ceará's Turnaround

When politicians in Ceará, the Northeastern state where I conducted my fieldwork, began adopting and promoting the health care reforms associated with the SUS, they did not claim to be improving Brazil's welfare state. Instead they touted these programs as replacing the much older system of patronage that dominated the Northeast for generations. In 2003 Fortaleza's secretary of health commented in a radio interview at the Universidade Federal do Ceará, "Health institutions used to be run by the mayors. Now with small councils in the communities, people are more involved [in health care matters], so they start demanding things."[6] The secretary was referring to the system of unequal exchanges and dependencies pervasive in Ceará in which mayors of small towns would often run municipal dispensaries where the rural poor could avail themselves of medical care in return for the appropriate vote. As I discuss in greater detail later in the book, Ceará's politicians and medical professionals repeatedly stressed to me that they were interested in a transition in the understanding of health care from a favor to a right.

International coverage of several innovative health care programs that Ceará adopted in the wake of the new health care reforms also drew attention to the erosion of state patronage and aristocratic privilege. Among the publications that touted Ceará's advances were *Newsweek*, *The Economist*, the *Christian Science Monitor*, and the *New York Times*. Carefully avoiding any mention of the country's landmark transition to a rights-based model of health care, these articles commended instead Ceará's sudden turnaround from an impoverished, paternalistic Northeastern state to a model of good governance intent on replacing networks of patronage with merit-based employment and educational opportunities. The reporters of these articles saw the shift toward "good governance" as enabling Ceará to move from the near-bottom to close to the top of Brazil's twenty-six states in terms of child-health indicators such as vaccinations, duration of breast-feeding, and child visits to pediatricians.

In extolling the moral virtues of vanquishing a corrupt regime, the articles explicitly celebrated the neoliberal political policies that were enacted to support Ceará's extensive health care reforms in the form of public-private partnerships. An article in the *New York Times*, for example, describes Ceará's development formula as "an aggressive attack on social ills paired with an equally aggressive courtship of private investors."[7] In the same article the reporter lauds the glamorous new Fortaleza, already evident by the mid-1990s, that went from a "northeastern dust bowl, with nothing to export but its population of workers" to a "beachfront city, full of European tourists and foreign investors, imported cars and a thriving fashion industry." I witnessed this transformation of Fortaleza firsthand; over the span of 1998–2009, during which I conducted fieldwork, every visit seemed to land me in a glitzier, ever more gentrified city with a wealthier and more entitled citizenry.

Although some of the newfound wealth seeped into the favela in ways that I track within this book, patronage and dependency have continued to dominate social life in the favela. Politicians made hopeful claims that the new regime of democratic and political rights would sweep away such *instituições antiquadas* (antiquated institutions), but older residents I knew in Pirambu continued to describe their social and economic superiors in terms of being *bons patrões* (good bosses) or *maus patrões* (unreliable or malevolent bosses). *Bons patrões*, depicted as kind, just, and generous, were carefully cultivated despite the potential of civil rights to directly provide the very forms of protection they sought from their superiors.[8]

Reciprocity among family members, friends, and neighbors also dominated the tempo of life in the favela. Household goods, food, medicine, and acts of care circulate continuously between homes in Pirambu. Contributions are solicited for residents in desperate straits, and sharing good fortune is expected. I rarely heard residents suggest that they had too little to be able to give to someone else who might need it more, and this ethic is one of the few that I observed transmitted unfailingly between generations.

In the domain of health, both patronage and reciprocity continue to structure social practice. A sick uncle might persuade his niece to contact the family who employs her as a maid to see if they have connections at a certain hospital. The neighbor of an ailing single mother will start a collection for medications, bus fare, and child care, not stopping until the need is met. The new health care system is intended to disrupt this older model of seeking care—by authorizing the pursuit of health as an inherent right belonging to each citizen rather than a product of social interactions mediated by one's position in society or in a local community. As a result, community residents confronted a health care system rooted in an ideology of individualized human rights layered on top of a social life deeply embedded in older systems of patronage and reciprocity and a neoliberal economic context that celebrated market exchange and individuals' abilities to fulfill their own needs and interests. Depictions of how residents navigated these multiple, overlapping, and often contradictory doctrines form the core of this book.

That Which Is Taken for Granted

When I arrived in Pirambu for the first time in 1998, it took me a long time to identify the public health care clinics that dotted the favela as places people went regularly for care and assistance. Part of this had to do with how seamlessly they blended in with the commercial and residential buildings on the streets. Low-slung, often without any formal placards announcing their purpose, health care clinics in Pirambu rarely stood out. But my initial inattention to the clinics also had to do with the way residents seemed to make little of the relatively robust network of neighborhood clinics. Nor did they appear startled that although getting their children through secondary school was often a dubious proposition, they could attend neighborhood clinics and even specialty hospitals without paying fees. It was this nonchalance, though, that eventually did attract my attention.

In *Outline of a Theory of Practice* (1977), Pierre Bourdieu uses the term "doxa" to denote that which is taken for granted in any particular society.[9] Doxa, according to Bourdieu, is the experience by which the natural and social world appear as self-evident or, as he succinctly puts it, what "goes without saying because it comes without saying" (167). In Pirambu, the existence of public health care clinics was largely taken for granted and appeared self-evident to residents. It was only when I started asking older residents who had been involved in the social movements of decades past to describe how the health care clinics had come about that I began to recognize the origins of the clinics as decidedly not self-evident and to learn about the extensive social and political activism required to bring them into existence.

Part of what most interests me with regard to health care reform in Ceará is the doxa that was created in its implementation and those that it replaced. Sean Brotherton, a medical anthropologist, has described this process in Cuba; he notes that "the socialist health care doxa has saturated people's everyday lives and mundane practices, producing state-fostered expectations and feelings of entitlement of particular forms of biomedical health care" (2012, 6).

But we can think of examples closer to home: the slow and uneven process of persuading Americans that smoking is bad for them or that seat belts must be worn while driving or that taking one's child to the doctor for immunizations is an important and even necessary part of parenting. All of these initiatives require not just political will and public implementation but a change in doxa, in people's attitudes about how they could and should behave and consequently in how they comport themselves. The success, I would argue, of any one of these public health campaigns required that they become a normalized, unremarkable part of everyday life, that they become "embodied," to use an anthropological term.

Fully realized health care reform requires a similar shift in doxa, as was explicitly recognized by health care officials in Ceará. While ushering in the reforms that accompanied the 1988 declaration of health care as a human right, administrators and state politicians in Ceará talked about the ways people would have to think anew about health care, as a right, not as a favor, or in terms of prevention instead of medical cures. But what these officials were not necessarily prepared for was the rapid commodification of medical services in Brazil that was exploding as the reforms were being implemented. These newly commodified and privatized health care services were increasingly attractive to a younger, consumer-oriented generation in the favela who aspired to services like dental care, caesarian sections, and private health care plans.

Thus, just as health care officials were working to build a doxa rooted in ideals of human rights, community participation, and preventive medicine, younger citizens living in the favela were beginning to pursue a vision of health care that revolved around notions of consumer freedom, individual choice, and self-enhancement. In documenting this clash of ideals and aspirations, I hope to contribute to a rich body of anthropological scholarship in Brazil that recognizes the extent to which medical services have become a key indicator of social difference among the urban poor (Béhague, Gonçalves, and Dias da Costa 2002; Biehl 2005, 2007; Edmonds 2004, 2007, 2010; McCullum 2005; Sanabria 2010).

To attend to this broad set of concerns I use descriptions of medical decision making, or what is known as health-seeking behavior, to capture changing expectations among Pirambu's residents about what health care could and should be and more broadly about what responsibility the state of Ceará or the city of Fortaleza has to its poorest citizens. I understand medical decision making to be a form of social reproduction; from the perspective of residents of Pirambu, various forms of medical care and treatment and of types of political participation around health care propose genuinely different accounts of personal identity and morality (Brodwin 1996). Thus when residents decide to seek private medical care instead of going to a local public clinic, ignore invitations to health care council meetings, or activate networks of patronage in order to access public medical care, they are engaging in acts of self-definition that reproduce individual ideas about health, community, belonging, and exclusion but also structural forms such as the levels of social class in the favela and the two-tiered health care system in which they are enmeshed.

Organization

A Right to Health is organized into two parts. In chapters 1 and 2 I describe the historical emergence of categories—democracy, citizenship, preventive medicine, public health, and participation—that constitute contemporary social life in Pirambu. In chapters 3 through 6 I investigate specific examples of health care reform, medical decision making, and community activism in the context of intergenerational tension in Pirambu.

In chapter 1 I describe how residents of Pirambu came to understand themselves as citizens of Fortaleza and to speak about their social and economic aspirations as civil rights, including the right to accessible health care. I contrast this historical account of citizenship in Pirambu with descriptions of how the practice of citizenship is being reformulated by a younger generation in the favela. In chapter 2 I trace the relationship between welfare assistance and the poor, describing how public health became a goal of the Brazilian state, the emergence of the public and private health care sectors in Ceará, and the local social movements that helped to extend health care to peripheral communities around Fortaleza.

In chapters 3 and 4, respectively, I examine two programs that arose as a result of the health care reforms in Fortaleza: democratic councils designed to involve a broad array of citizens in the creation and implementation of new health care practices and Farmácia Viva, a public health program devoted to ensuring the correct and scientific use of traditional medicine. I use an examination of the health councils and Farmácia Viva to highlight tensions and shifts in Pirambu in concepts such as participation, health, and preventive medicine.

In chapters 5 and 6 I explore the generational divide in the practices and discourses that have surrounded medical decision making in Pirambu. I suggest that paradoxically the universal right to health guaranteed in the 1988 constitution is being undermined by a new generation of young favela residents for whom health care appears to be neither a favor nor a right but rather something that, in its privatized form, has become an aspiration. In my conclusion I analyze contemporary social movements in the favela that have shifted away from protests directed at achieving social equity and toward expanding individual freedom to exercise choice. These shifts in the practice and form of social activism help to explain some of the contradictions observed throughout the book in the history and current unfolding of health care reform in Ceará.

Notes on Method

I lived in the community of Pirambu from October 1998 through August 1999. In the fall of 2001 I spent another three months in the community, and I returned again for two-month periods in the summers of 2005, 2007, and 2009. The decade span of fieldwork visits allowed me to track shifts that I saw emerging there in terms of how residents were defining themselves, their political views, and their health care practices as well as broader changes in the community such as how social movements were evolving. Repeated visits to the field enabled me to form close friendships within several groups of residents, which helped me to develop something closer to an insider's perspective on the favela than might have otherwise been available to me.

Several additional circumstances were important to how I conducted my field research. During my first period of fieldwork I lived with an older woman, Isabella Ribeiro, and her thirteen-year-old adopted daughter, Vera. Living in such close quarters with the same two people throughout the first part of my research meant that the world I got to know in the favela was, at least at first, largely their world. I came to know their friends and family members, I frequented their favorite markets and snack shops, and I visited the schools and religious institutions they attended. Although I broadened these experiences during the latter months of the first period of fieldwork and ultimately was able to sustain broader networks of relations in the favela, my research is unquestionably conditioned by the formation of these initial relationships.

I arrived in Pirambu under the direction of Adalberto Barreto, a psychiatrist and professor of social medicine at the Universidade Federal do Ceará who had spent nearly a decade advocating on behalf of the community and providing mental health services for its residents. My connection to Adalberto had several advantages. First, he was generally well liked within the community, and thus I was almost immediately accepted and looked after by the residents he knew in Pirambu. Second, Adalberto was extremely well connected to the medical community in Fortaleza, which made pursuing interviews with public health agents and government officials much easier than it might have been.

Finally, toward the end of my first period of fieldwork in Pirambu I met six young women friends from the neighborhood who took it upon themselves to rescue me from what was perceived as the very dour work of conducting interviews and following people around to their various medical appointments. Excursions to the mall and nearby beaches soon followed, and as I grew undoubtedly happier in daily life in the favela, I also came to understand more about the community in which I was living. Much of what I have written about an emerging, younger, and more upwardly mobile class in the favela is based on my interactions with this group of women and their extensive network of friends and family members. Though the daily practices and ideologies I observed within this milieu were not representative of "average" favela life, it was certainly a robust and increasingly vocal segment of Pirambu's population and serves as a reminder, as scholars who work in urban peripheral areas of Brazil have commented, that these communities are composed of multiple social and economic classes (Caldeira 2006; Holston 2008; Perlman 1976, 2010).

The bulk of the ethnographic data upon which I base this book is composed of the illness narratives, medical case studies, and life histories I collected during my fieldwork. The collection of these data required participant observation and intensive formal and informal interviews. Once I had lived in the community for several months and had come to know people on a more intimate basis, I asked if I might accompany them on future visits to doctors and clinics. I was rarely turned down, and the poverty and duress under which most residents of Pirambu suffer meant that there was rarely a shortage of opportunities to accompany someone to a clinic visit or to observe them in the midst of medical decision making. The case studies I compiled for this book are drawn from a total of approximately fifty such studies I collected during my multiple stays in Pirambu. Most people requested that their real names be used, and that is what I have done with the exception of several residents described in chapters 1 and 6 who requested that names of their choosing be used instead.

In addition to observing medical decision making and recording life histories of those involved in the decisions and of their immediate family members, I spent my time becoming acquainted with the public and private health care system of Fortaleza. On every trip to a hospital or medical clinic I made with a resident of Pirambu, I met with someone at the medical institution and would often return the next day or week for follow-up interviews. At Farmácia Viva, the focus of chapter 4, I conducted interviews with the program's staff and recorded observations I made at several of its clinics.

Fortaleza's political elite was small and accessible enough that I managed to speak with many people who worked at the top level of the city's health care delivery system. Living in the favela while I was conducting research meant that I was constantly traveling into Fortaleza from the same starting point as residents themselves. Though not an insider by any means, I believe I acquired an additional kind of knowledge by taking the same buses residents of Pirambu took, often arriving at interviews sweaty, tired, and uncomfortably thirsty and returning at night, descending from the bus back into the dense atmosphere of the favela.

The final data upon which I base this study are derived from the archival research I conducted about the history of Pirambu and the popular social movements out of which the favela and its social services emerged. I must stress that I was particularly fortunate in this endeavor in that Pirambu has an office, the Centro Popular de Pesquisa, Documentação e Comunicação (CPDOC), specifically devoted to the compiling of historical and statistical data about the favela. The office was small but contained reams of material about the community compiled by social historians, regional scholars, and students and professors from Fortaleza's two research universities. Most low-income communities do not have the benefits of such a detailed written history, and the center serves as a reminder of the high degree of external involvement in Pirambu as well as the self-consciousness and political awareness of many of its residents.

CHAPTER ONE

Pirambu: Historical and Contemporary
Accounts of Citizenship in a Favela

If you take the Grande Circular 2 due west from the city's old, baroque courthouse, now the nocturnal haunt of prostitutes, past the new Dragão do Mar cultural center and the crumbling Biblioteca Pública, over one of the city's few overpasses, and then down along the Avenida Presidente Castelo Branco, better known simply as Leste-Oeste (East-West), you will eventually end up in Pirambu. During the morning and evening rush hours the bus is crammed full of residents from Pirambu, many of whom work in downtown Fortaleza. As the bus grinds its way toward the favela, swaying under the weight of its visibly exhausted but still courteous passengers, it passes the meticulously restored Marina del Mar, a country club for Fortaleza's elite and a symbol of the city's growing grandeur. A hastily built sewage treatment plant sits, incongruously, just on the other side of the Marina del Mar, causing people to hold handkerchiefs over their mouths and roll their eyes at one another, though its smells differ little from those that invade the favela itself. Finally, the bus reaches a long row of densely built cinderblock homes, each no more than two stories high, interspersed with bakeries, pharmacies, cafés, churches, fruit and vegetable stands, clothing stores, and the occasional gas station, and flanked by looming billboards promoting an astounding array of commodities or, less often, public service announcements.

Pirambu is one of numerous favelas within the city of Fortaleza.[1] Its enviable location sprawling along the Atlantic coast less than two miles from downtown, its comparatively deep historical roots as a fishing community that originated in the 1850s, and its well-developed commercial and social service infrastructure set Pirambu apart from the city's other low-income neighborhoods. Extending along the ocean and the recently renovated Leste-Oeste, Pirambu has a population of more than forty thousand residents. It is the largest favela in Ceará and among the ten largest in all of Brazil.[2]

Home to some of the poorest among Fortaleza's 2.5 million residents,[3] Pirambu holds a prominent place in the social imaginations of the city's upper-class citizens. Over years of conducting interviews with middle- and upper-middle-class professionals in Fortaleza, I consistently heard Pirambu described as a dangerous, dirty, and troublesome area. Very occasionally I would meet someone who took the view that residents of the favela bore vestiges of a deeply romanticized version of Ceará's rural interior and were thus at odds with the urban squalor in which they now resided. But more often the portrayals were less hopeful; a city official said to me when I told her I was staying on the outskirts of Fortaleza, "This city has only one *bairro sofisticado* [upscale neighborhood]; the rest of the city is violent and full of poverty."

This view was most clearly enacted by the precautions I saw city officials and health professionals take when they needed to engage directly with the community. On these occasions, the professionals would arrive in large, expensive cars with tinted windows, driving as close to their destinations in the favela as possible despite the work it required to get their bulky cars through the narrow, cobbled alleyways. Once inside the favela, they traveled in pairs, kept their cell phones close at hand, and always left well before dark.

The forbidding, stereotyped descriptions of Pirambu overlook the community's long history of political and social engagement with the city of Fortaleza as well as the attendant transformation of that neighborhood from an impoverished fishing village into an urbanized, legal district with a full complement of social and commercial services. Pirambu was built up over seventy-plus years through the process of what James Holston and Teresa Caldeira have called "autoconstruction" (Holston 1991, Caldeira and Holston 2005). As Holston elaborates at length in his incisive ethnography on Brazilian citizenship (2008), autoconstruction is the experience by which Brazil's working classes moved to cities and built up the urban peripheries, creating a new form of civic participation and practice of citizenship rights in the process.

The paths trodden by residents of Pirambu to transform their neighborhood mirror those taken by favela residents in the southern city of São Paulo as described by Holston. In both cases, as residents slowly turned their fragile, one-story, wooden shacks into colorful, cinderblock, multistory dwellings, the peripheries became spaces of "alterna-

tive futures" (Holston 2008). In them, the very experience of organizing social movements, participating in consumer markets, and making
decisions about just what those new and improved houses should look
like convinced residents living on the margins of the city that they were
in fact worthy of the political and civic rights the city bestowed on its
wealthier citizens. As they articulated this transformation in their own
ideas of citizenship, Pirambu's residents went from having only occasional access to rights through limited political and civic recognition to
eventually being recognized as citizens who intrinsically bear the "right
to rights." A range of individual rights was legally enshrined in the 1988
Constituição da República Federativa do Brasil that included the provision stipulating that "health is a right of every individual and a duty of
the state."

Brazilian scholars have carefully traced the diverse segments of society—from intellectuals and health service researchers to worker organizations and political parties—involved in the social movements that
led up to the constitutional amendment conferring the right to health
(Dagnino 2007, Escorel 1999, Fleury 1997, Teixeira 1989). One of the
central arguments of this book is that a history of this process can also
be found in an urban peripheral neighborhood in Northeastern Brazil
where residents experimented with the idea of a "right to health" for
decades as it became embedded in their community. In the first part
of this chapter I describe the slow and deliberate process by which Pirambu's residents came to understand themselves as citizens of Fortaleza
whose economic and social aspirations could be understood in terms of
civil rights, including the right to health care, and in turn transformed
their community from an illegally settled fishing village into a highly
urbanized, legal neighborhood.

What is striking about the history of Pirambu is that while prior
scholarship has tended to date the emergence of rights-based language
among favela dwellers in Brazil to the 1970s (Holston 2008, Scheper-
Hughes 1992), I have found newspaper articles that offer clear evidence
of residents using rights-based arguments to demand social services
from the city of Fortaleza as early as the 1940s. This finding highlights
the extremely localized nature of the emergence of citizen subjectivity
and the importance of analyzing this process in multiple and diverse lo-
calities (Forment 2003, Win 1989). Later in the chapter I give several
ethnographic examples of the practice of citizenship among residents in
Pirambu in order to demonstrate the variations, tensions, and explicit
contradictions in contemporary forms of citizen subjectivity.

The Emergence of Rights-Based Claims to Citizenship in Pirambu

I think our making the history of Pirambu was an important moment for us residents of this long-suffering, exploited neighborhood that served as a guinea pig . . . Since the bourgeoisie has it all . . . [and] puts its greatest individuals in the history books, why can't we workers, who built the world, also have our own history told, written, televised?

—JOSÉ MARIA TABOSA, PIRAMBU RESIDENT, 1999

The community of Pirambu began not as a favela but as a small fishing village in the mid-1800s composed primarily of people who had fled rural inland areas of Ceará during the droughts that periodically ravage the state. Its residents named their community after the fish known as *Pirambu* commonly found in the Atlantic waters off the coast of Fortaleza, and they made their living by selling fish at the city's local markets. Even today, Pirambu's beaches are lined with elegant variations of the traditional Northeastern fishing boats known as *jangadas* and in the early mornings are swarming with residents for whom fishing remains a primary livelihood.

The community's tranquil origins were disrupted when in 1862 a cholera epidemic broke out in Fortaleza, causing eleven thousand deaths. To help contain the outbreak, city officials built a small hospital and cemetery on the outskirts of town near Pirambu. Those who were infected with cholera were sent to stay in the hospital; those who died of the disease were buried in the cemetery (Gonçalves da Costa 1995, 11). A few years later a leprosy colony was relocated to Pirambu, and lepers were sent there to live apart from the rest of the population.

By the early 1900s the city had adopted a formal policy of banning the sick and the poor as well as more obvious eyesores such as prostitutes and beggars from the more prosperous eastern zone (Zona Leste) of Fortaleza. The western zone of the city (Zona Oeste), where poor neighborhoods such as Pirambu were located, came to house these unwanted populations. City officials claimed they were following hygiene models then popular in southern Brazilian cities like Rio de Janeiro that encouraged the removal of the sick and the poor to outlying areas to prevent the spread of deadly epidemics. In fact, the policies helped institutionalize profound inequalities in the distribution of the city's resources, providing neighborhoods in the eastern zone with water, electricity, garbage disposal, and public schools while completely neglecting neighborhoods in the western zone (Gonçalves da Costa 1995).

The bifurcation of the city intensified in 1932 when settlement camps were established in the western zone to house rural migrants who continued flooding into the city to escape the ravages of drought. Business leaders in the city also had begun to build manufacturing plants on the outer edges of the western zone to produce commodities such as soap and leather. Migrants who were newly arrived to the city and looking for work quickly filled these plants. Thus, by the late 1930s the western zone of Fortaleza had come to represent perversion, sickness, death, and industrial pollution in the imaginations of Fortaleza's more affluent classes, and these morbid associations stigmatized the residents who lived there.

Newspaper articles of the period confirmed the poor living conditions of Pirambu's residents and further conflated the physical conditions with the residents themselves. The headline of an article in 1932 proclaims "O acampamento dos flagelados no Pirambu" (The settlement of the poor in Pirambu) and goes on to decry both the diseases and inhospitable living conditions endemic to the area and the undesirables who made it their home—prostitutes, thieves, and beggars (*O Povo*, April 11, 1932). More than a decade later, articles continued to sound similar themes, as did this one in *O Democrata* of February 3, 1948: "A praia do Pirambu está transformada num antro de prostitutas, bêbados e ladrões" (The beach of Pirambu is transformed into a lair of prostitutes, drunks, and thieves).

The popular perception of the residents as undesirables was reinforced by their formal relationship to the city of Fortaleza; from the community's inception and up through the 1930s, Pirambu's residents were systematically denied access to political, civil, and social citizenship. Despite their contributions to the city's growing manufacturing sector, residents were technically ineligible to vote in local and national elections,[4] join local labor unions, or hold titles to the lots on which they had built their houses. Thus as a whole they lived as squatters, with their births, deaths, and marriages unrecorded by city officials and without access to schools, medical clinics, public transportation, or other city services (Farias 1997).

Political and economic aspirations began to develop among Pirambu's residents as the community's population dramatically increased during the 1940s. Starting in the mid-1930s, rural-to-urban migration brought thousands of Northeasterners to the southern industrial cities of São Paulo, Rio de Janeiro, and Belo Horizonte and a rapidly increasing stream of migrants from inland Ceará to Fortaleza.

The pattern of urbanization in Fortaleza followed that of the Northeastern region as a whole. In 1920 the city had a population of 78,500. By 1940 the population jumped to 180,200, an increase of 130 percent. In 1950 the population reached 270,200, representing another 50 percent increase. And by 1960 the total population of the city reached 514,800, marking another 91 percent increase in one decade (R. Brooks 1972, 143). The major population increases in Pirambu paralleled the city's growth, transforming a community of 8,000 to 10,000 residents in the 1930s into one of 40,000 residents by 1960. The great majority of these new residents were migrants from rural areas of Ceará (Ceará 1967, Gonçalves da Costa 1995).

The growth in population was accompanied by a marked increase in residents' demands on the city of Fortaleza to improve their living conditions. A survey of Fortaleza's three major newspapers—*O Democrata*, *O Povo*, and *Gazeta de Notícias*—between 1940, when social protests were first reported, to 1964, the start of the military dictatorship, demonstrates that a wide range of economic and social aspirations motivated Pirambu's residents to political action.

An article in *O Democrata* of August 4, 1953, begins with the headline and subhead "A pobreza trabalha muito, ganha pouco e come menos. Nossa reportagem ouve donas de casa, as que mais sofrem com a crescente alta do custo de vida—Revolta geral contra o aumento do sabão" (The poor work a lot, earn little, and eat less. Our report listens to housewives, those who suffer most from the increasingly high cost of living—General revolt against the rise [in the price] of soap). The women interviewed for the article complained about the high prices of everyday food articles and wanted prices of necessary foodstuffs to be kept below a maximum price.

Another issue that roiled Pirambu's residents during the early 1950s was the constant rise in transportation costs. A headline in *O Democrata* of October 10, 1949, declared, "Nem um centavo a mais para os tubarões dos transportes! Vibrante manifesto da Sociedade de Defesa dos Moradores do Pirambu contra a exploração dos empresários de ônibus" (Not one cent more for the transportation sharks! Vibrant demonstration of the Society of the Defense of Inhabitants of Pirambu against the exploitation by bus company owners).

Newspaper articles described the broad swath of issues Pirambu residents wanted the city to address over the years. An article in *O Democrata* of June 13, 1958, bears the headline "Pirambu: 30 mil habitantes. O bairro luta com a falta d'água—O problema da higiene—falta de luz e de calçamento" (Pirambu: 30,000 inhabitants. The neighborhood fights against lack of water, problems of hygiene, lack of electricity and street paving). These issues, along with concerns about land rights, education, and access to medical facilities, recur in newspaper accounts of protests in Pirambu starting in the 1940s and continuing through the early 1960s.

A striking aspect of the news articles and other documents I reviewed is that from very early on, residents understood the social and economic aspirations they were articulating as rights of citizenship and the city government as responsible for fulfilling their ideals. An April 2, 1949, headline in the *Gazeta do Ceará* reads, "Os moradores do Pirambu não cederão os seus direitos" (The residents of Pirambu won't cede their rights). The article discusses residents' unwillingness to give up their land to government officials who were attempting to expropriate it for a planned harbor. An article in *O Democrata* of September 8, 1949, shows residents making a more direct accusation of the city government: "O governo quer matar o povo de fome!" (The government wants to kill the people by hunger!).

A decade later, the *Gazeta de Notícias* of May 25, 1960, announced, "Pirambu vem ao centro: quer ajuda para ser menos pobre!" (Pirambu comes downtown: it wants help to be less poor!). Finally, in what would be the culminating protest of the era, in 1962 the Grande Marcha do Pirambu (Grand March of Pirambu) took place. Somewhere between twenty thousand and forty thousand people marched to the Palácio do Governo to demand recognition of their neighborhood, delivery of city services and, most importantly, legal titles to their land. During the march, residents of Pirambu carried banners that read "Nós Cremos No Amor" (We believe in love) and demanded specific services from the state. They shouted, "Queremos escola para os nossos filhos!" (We want school for our children!) and "Queremos saúde para nossas famílias!" (We want health for our families!). They asserted their desire to be recognized as citizens of the city, crying "Somos parte de Fortaleza!" (We are part of Fortaleza!). And, in perhaps the most self-conscious recognition that belonging to a political entity entitles its citizens to certain rights, residents asserted "O Estado é para o homem, e não o homem para o estado!" (The state is to serve the people, and not the people [to serve] the state!) (in Gonçalves da Costa 1995, 22).

Political activism from 1940 to 1964 came in fits and starts but remained startlingly consistent in its central message: residents aspired to a broad array of city services and resources and viewed themselves as entitled to these assets because they were already part of Fortaleza and thus worthy beneficiaries of its growing prosperity.

Political and Civil Achievements

The ongoing protests and marches of the 1940s, 1950s, and early 1960s resulted in an impressive array of achievements for residents of Pirambu, in terms of both the formal political rights they were able to secure and the dramatic increase in social services and infrastructure to the community they realized. One of the most important accomplishments came when residents of Pirambu gained legal titles to their land in 1962. Up until that time, they suffered from threats by businessmen who wanted to build factories or other industrial plants on their land. Under the guidance and strong encouragement of a Catholic priest, Hélio Campos, who had arrived in Fortaleza several years earlier, residents began to resist expulsion from their homes and participate in organized marches to the governor's palace in Fortaleza to demand recognition of their community.

According to older residents with whom I spoke, Padre Campos was instrumental in helping to organize the 1962 Grande Marcha do Pirambu. He urged them to draw attention to the illegality of denying favela dwellers land titles. This time they were successful, and on May 25, 1962, Law 1.058 was signed by the governor of Ceará, Virgílio Távora, officially declaring 427 acres to belong to residents of Pirambu and calling for an increase of city services in the area (Gonçalves da Costa 1995, 23).

Following the march, Pirambu became the pioneer of the Movimento Social Urbano de Fortaleza, which demanded more social services for poor communities throughout Fortaleza. Over the next several years, dozens of community organizations were formed in Pirambu, and a majority of the neighborhood's homes were supplied with electricity and potable water (Gonçalves da Costa 1995, 23). By the early 1960s, a fair proportion of the civil rights to which Pirambu residents had long aspired had been achieved: they now held titles to their land; birth, death, and marriage certificates were becoming more routine; electricity, roads, and plumbing were extended to their community; and schools, day care centers, and small businesses were springing up all around the favela.

The developments point to a relationship that had been emerging between Fortaleza's poorest residents and city politicians since the late 1940s. The explicit hierarchy that had defined the city's relationship to its peripheral communities for generations was being challenged by Pirambu residents as their increasing demands encouraged city politicians to compete for their votes. Newspaper articles as far back as the 1940s show that multiple city council members visited Pirambu to demonstrate their awareness of the community's plight: "2 vereadores de Prestes amanhã no Pirambu" (Two city council members of [Mayor] Prestes tomorrow in Pirambu) (*O Democrata*, August 2, 1948); and "Alísio Mamede falará à noite de hoje no Pirambu, Parangabussú, e São João do Tauape. Em contato com o povo os candidatos da Frente Democrática debaterão com as massas os seus mais importantes problemas" (Alísio Mamede will speak tonight in Pirambu, Parangabussú, e São João do Tauape. In contact with the people the candidates of the Frente Democrática [Democratic Front] will debate with the masses their most important problems) (*O Democrata*, September 11, 1950). The latter article discusses the increasing attention poor communities like Pirambu were receiving from city council members eager to build up their constituencies.

James Holston makes clear in his account of favela residents in São Paulo that the kind of subjectivity that developed under these circumstances, in which residents experienced having their needs met by participating directly in neighborhood associations and making community-level demands of politicians, was quite different from the consciousness that arose under the earlier client-patron relationships in which the poor were entitled to only a minimum form of social assistance and charity in exchange for their votes (2008, 248). This older form of social belonging, typical of the early years in Pirambu and writ large in famous Brazilian texts such as Gilberto Freyre's 1933 opus, *Casa grande e senzala* (translated as *The Masters and the Slaves*), is often associated with a meek and passive spirit and an unwillingness to improve one's condition.

But depictions of Pirambu's residents found in newspaper articles and oral testimonials of the 1940s through the early 1960s do not conform to the stereotypical images of the Brazilian poor as a mass of largely ignorant folk stuck in rural traditions and subdued by wealthy patrons. Rather, they demonstrate that well before the onset of the military dictatorship, residents of Pirambu had become articulate and demanding residents of Fortaleza who achieved recognition from the city as they paid their taxes and became property holders and consumers in neighborhood and city marketplaces. As various scholars remind us (Biehl 2005, Caldeira 2006, Holston 2008, Scheper-Hughes 1992), it cannot be suggested that patron-client relationships disappeared completely or that favela residents' lives were not still defined by hierarchy, patronage, and inequality. I show quite emphatically later in this chapter and throughout the remainder of the book that older forms of social belonging as well as newer forms of social inequality have continued to shape residents' lives. Nonetheless, by the early 1960s residents of Pirambu successfully achieved a possible alternative mode of being. In "making the history of Pirambu" they made themselves into sometime citizens of the city in which they resided.

From Military Dictatorship to Political Democracy

The onset of the military dictatorship in 1964 had an almost immediate effect on the progress of social justice in the favela. The few extant written accounts of the effect on Pirambu stress that from the start of the dictatorship the Catholic Church was strongly discouraged from participating in progressive movements throughout Fortaleza's peripheral communities and that consequently social movements in Pirambu began to shut down (Brito 1996, Gonçalves da Costa 1995, Silva 1999). Historical accounts of Ceará confirm that progressive and popular movements in Fortaleza suffered severe repression under the dictatorship. The popular historian Aírton Farias has noted (1997) that in 1970 the newly formed paramilitary Movimento Anti-Comunista (MAC, Anti-Communist Movement) conducted several explicit attacks on leftist organizations, including one on the Diretório Central dos Estudantes (DCE, Students Central Executive Committee) of the Universidad Federal do Ceará. Newspaper articles I surveyed from the dictatorship era no longer contained reports of protests and social organizing in the city's peripheral communities and became largely silent with regard to progress in them.

In contrast to these dramatic events, the majority of older residents whom I asked about life under the dictatorship rarely spoke about the era in vivid terms. "Things went on," one told me, and "life continued just the same." A woman said to me, "Well, we were poor then. We were still very poor." Only residents who were deeply involved in the organizing and social protests of the pre-dictatorship period recalled specific details about the subsequent era. Several of them told me that Padre

Campos was prohibited from conducting services in Pirambu in 1968 and was transferred to the state of Maranhão in 1969.

Written historical accounts of the favela confirm these events and show that by 1970 two new priests were sent to minister to Pirambu's residents (Brito 1996, Silva 1999). The priests were under the leadership of the new archbishop of Fortaleza, Aloísio Lorsheider. In an unusual turn for the era, Lorsheider emerged as a progressive leader who, despite the dictatorship, cautiously encouraged the priests of poor congregations to return to issues of education, health, housing, and employment.

Thus in the early 1970s, although there were still major restrictions on social movements at the national level, social and political activism began to reemerge in peripheral communities in Fortaleza (Brito 1996, Silva 1999). In Pirambu, residents continued to make demands on the city for paved roads, electricity, and basic sanitation (Gonçalves da Costa 1995, 31). And important social service organizations such as the Centro Educacional Moema Távora (an educational center that offered a range of classes for children in the favela) and Conselhos Comunitários (an entity that encouraged leadership and social networks in the community) as well as a medical clinic, Maternidade Nossa Senhora das Graças, were opened in Pirambu during this time as well (ibid., 29).

During the 1980s, with the gradual return to civilian government, several organizations were created at the federal level whose resources eventually made their way to Pirambu. The Secretaria Especial de Habitação e Ação Comunitária (Special Department of Housing and Community Action) developed programs to improve life in the country's favelas, among them the Programa Nacional do Leite (PNL, National Milk Program), Programa do Mutirão Habitacional (Community Homebuilding Program), and Fala Favela (Speak, Favela), now a nationwide organization to help favela dwellers articulate their needs and concerns (Gonçalves da Costa 1995, 41). Pirambu's residents asserted that they had benefited in particular from the Programa do Mutirão Habitacional, designed to encourage joint government and community participation in the construction of new houses in low-income neighborhoods. In 1987 the program began delivering housing materials and organizing Pirambu residents into cooperative work groups. By 1989 residents had collectively built 2,267 new houses in the favela (Gonçalves da Costa 1995, 41).

Politics had opened up considerably in Ceará since the start of the Brazilian dictatorship, and in 1985 Maria Luiza Fontenele of the Partido dos Trabalhadores (PT, Workers Party) was elected mayor of Fortaleza. Several residents with whom I spoke about the final years of the dictatorship said Fontenele redirected politicians' attention to the issues of education and health care for favela dwellers, and residents recalled hearing their concerns regularly addressed on the local radio and television stations for the first time in the community's history.

In 1988, under civilian President José Sarney, the Brazilian government drafted a new constitution that granted an extensive set of fundamental political and civil rights to all citizens. The new constitution strengthened safeguards against state crimes as well as treason. The constitution established forms of direct popular participation besides regular voting, such as plebiscite, referendum, and the possibility of ordinary citizens proposing new laws.

Again, James Holston stresses the connection between these significant achievements at the federal, now constitutional level and the decades-long political struggles and accomplishments of favela dwellers. His argument is worth quoting at length:

> This mobilization turned the insurgent citizens of the urban peripheries into key protagonists in a national struggle over the nature of the new charter for Brazilian society. . . . Their objective was to insure that it embody their experiences—their conflicts, needs, rights, and perspectives as the modern urban working classes of Brazil—as a basic source of substantive rights and social justice. Along with their compatriots in the countryside, their battle was, in essence, for the democratic imagination of the Constitutional Assembly (Assembléia Constituinte, 1986–1988) elected by direct popular vote. (2008, 250)

The foregoing discussion in this chapter should lend weight to Holston's argument: residents of urban poor communities like Pirambu were not abruptly bestowed with democratic rights but had in fact been working toward them for most of their lives.

Despite these achievements, multiple authors have stressed the entanglements of traditional and clientelistic political structures, special-treatment rationales, and new forms of urban citizenship that have been simultaneously present in Brazil and must be negotiated, to different effects, by wealthy and low-income residents alike (Caldeira 2006, Goldstein 2003, Holston 2008, Scheper-Hughes 1992). In Ceará, as throughout Brazil, the negotiations were deeply shaped by the concomitant shift of political administrators to neoliberal economic and development policies (Dagnino 2007).

To illustrate the effects neoliberalism has had on Fortaleza's economic and social life, it is instructive to look at the example of Tasso Jereissati, who was elected governor in 1986 on the promise that he would combat misery and paternalism but also with the explicit understanding that he would open up the state to foreign investment and liberalize its financial sectors (Farias 1997). By certain standards, the economic reforms and incentive programs Jereissati implemented were hugely successful. From 1985 to 1993 the gross domestic product of Ceará rose by 50 percent, the largest increase in all of Brazil (*Veja*, December 1, 1993, 91). International investments boomed during the early 1990s, and six Taiwanese manufacturing companies invested a hundred million dollars in Fortaleza businesses. As a direct result of this type of investment, two hundred upscale franchise stores opened in Fortaleza in the early 1990s, while more than two hundred apartment buildings, two thousand office buildings, and one thousand stores went into construction (ibid., 92).

Fortaleza's success in acquiring the trappings of a thriving, cosmopolitan city encouraged state officials to seek to develop the state's tourism industry. Urban improvement projects were planned throughout the city, and particular attention was paid to enhancing the city's long, sparkling coastline. As a result of these endeavors, Fortaleza's economic indexes show that between 1993 and 1995 tourist visits increased significantly. In 1993 the four-star hotels in Fortaleza had a median occupancy rate during the year of about 60 percent; by 1995 occupancy had grown to 70 percent. The rates have continued to climb, and the tourist industry as a whole has come to play an increasingly important role in the state's economy.

One of the most striking aspects of the economic development that took place in Fortaleza during the 1990s is how rapidly it transpired. I vividly remember landing for the first time in Fortaleza in 1997, for language training, at what I considered the typical small, tropical city airport; it was a tiny, open-air structure crowded with relatives and assorted hagglers. When I returned to conduct fieldwork just one year later, I found myself landing at Fortaleza's new international airport. The airport's space-age architecture, air-conditioned corridors, and wide array of retail shops and restaurants had much in common with the new malls I was also soon to discover on the edges of the city. Though still rare, the buildings offered lavish examples of the kind of city that its officials hoped Fortaleza would become.

Throughout the time I was conducting fieldwork in Pirambu, the city of Fortaleza continued to invest money and resources in urban renewal projects that primarily benefited Fortaleza's elite and the tourists who came to sample the state's beaches. I saw the opening in 1999 of the Dragão do Mar (Sea Dragon), a beautiful, modern cultural center in downtown Fortaleza with an art-house movie theater, a lovely café, a planetarium, and a museum with Ceará folk art as well as a small modern art collection. The center is composed of a set of graceful, open-air buildings—forming arches like a dragon's back above older city structures—in an area that was brought back to life with the opening of restaurants, bars, and nightclubs. The more time I spent in Pirambu and elsewhere in Fortaleza, the more I realized it was not just the residents of the favela who were looking toward the future; dreams, both modest and grandiose, were what fueled Ceará's capital city.

Aírton Farias's account of Ceará's economic growth during the 1990s emphasizes the social and economic inequalities that have plagued the state since its inception. Power and wealth remain concentrated in the hands of a few, and despite the accolades that Ceará has won for its statewide health care programs, in general government officials have paid much greater attention to generating foreign investment and enhancing Ceará's commercial districts than they have to social welfare issues. Farias notes that in 1996 the state government spent nearly four times the amount of money on commercial ventures that it did on social ones (1997, 266).

The imbalance in expenditures did not go unnoticed by leaders in Pirambu. Padre Francisco, a priest in Pirambu's largest Catholic church, told me during an interview in the summer of 2000, "These last four years, when unemployment has grown so much, are the worst that I've seen in the favela—and that includes the dictatorship era. The impact of unemployment is huge. They keep talking about 'globalization,' but what's it going to do? Who's it going to help?"

Contemporary Experiments in Negotiating Citizenship

The following ethnographic examples describe events that I saw unfold during the course of repeated fieldwork visits of 1998–2009. They illustrate the complicated mixture of political alliances, legal structures, and family networks that Pirambu's residents must negotiate in the pursuit of mundane as well as more elevated aspirations, and they highlight the personal and moral frameworks residents use to interpret these experiences. The first example follows the struggles of a woman I knew well, Isabella Ribeiro, to secure housing for her only daughter, Vera.

Keeping House

Maria Isabella Ribeiro was fifty-two when I met her in 1998. A practical, hardworking, and slightly cautious woman, her primary concern at the time was the welfare of her adopted daughter, Vera. Isabella's life trajectory was, in many ways, exemplary of generations of Northeasterners who had grown up in the rural interior of their states and moved to city centers as young adults. Isabella was born in 1946 on a small *fazenda* (ranch) named São João Acaraú near the coastal town of Jericoacoara. Isabella's father worked as a sharecropper on the *fazenda*, growing cotton, cassava, and enough subsistence crops to feed his family. When she was six, her mother died of an infection acquired during the birth of her fourth child. Her father remarried almost immediately and moved with his new wife to another *fazenda* in the south of the state, leaving his four children with his former mother-in-law, who lived on a bit of land nearby.

In 1959, as part of the mass migrations that brought millions of people from the interior to Brazil's large cities, Isabella's older brother moved to Fortaleza to help support the family. Three years later, at the age of sixteen, Isabella joined him. When she moved to Fortaleza she lived briefly in Pirambu with her brother. However, he soon became unemployed, and Isabella decided it would be easier for both of them if she moved in with their aunt and uncle who lived just outside of the favela in a lower-middle-class neighborhood. Here she began working in a pharmacy, starting out as a low-level assistant and eventually filling complicated pharmaceutical orders on her own.

Isabella often described this era of her life to me, the years from 1965 until her marriage in 1988, in glowing detail: "I was living on my own in the city. I had a *bom patrão* [good boss]. He was kind to me and took care of everyone who worked in the shop. I was making a regular salary that came with health and retirement benefits [courtesy of Getúlio Vargas's social security program], and I had a little extra to spend each month on a movie or to give to my aunt and uncle." She stated unequivocally that this was one of the "truly good parts" of her life, when "many things seemed within reach."

When I asked if she had taken part in the protests that dominated Pirambu at the time, she admitted that she had not. "I didn't think of my-self as poor," she explained. "I could read, I had a stable job with benefits, and I was working toward saving up for a house of my own." She further described herself as a "boa trabalhadora" (a good worker) and thus as someone who would be able to improve her conditions well beyond what her parents had achieved. As it happened, these years would mark the last time Isabella would consider herself a part of the upwardly mobile working class.

At the age of forty-two Isabella met and married a man to whom her co-worker at the pharmacy had introduced her. Her new husband, Fernando da Silva, was a self-made man who had worked all his life in construction and saved up a considerable sum of money. Isabella spent the first year of her marriage helping him move around Fortaleza from house to house, each one slightly less distinguished than the one before it due to her husband's increasing gambling debts. Hoping that he would reform, Isabella convinced her husband to move to Boa Vista, the small town in southern Ceará where her father lived. Within a year, however, Isabella realized that her husband would remain a drunkard and, more deleteriously, had gambled away nearly their entire combined savings.

Her strict Catholic upbringing and her own deeply held religious convictions would not allow her to seek a divorce, but in 1991 Isabella separated permanently from her husband. Though she admitted that she was weighed down by the disappointment of her broken marriage, Isabella made clear that her recollections of this period were brightened by her decision to adopt Vera.

Isabella's half-sister, Maria Clara, who had been living in Pirambu, gave birth to her sixth child some three years earlier and was struggling with taking care of all of her children in addition to working at a nearby *caju* (cashew) processing factory. When she learned that Isabella was longing for a child but not able to carry one of her own, she offered to give her Vera. Isabella said she gladly accepted her sister's offer and decided to return to Fortaleza permanently.

Initially, Isabella and three-year-old Vera moved in with Maria Clara's mother, who also lived in Pirambu. Her long-term plan, however, was to buy a small house in the area to finally fulfill her dream of homeownership. In 1994 Isabella purchased a small, cinderblock house from a local businessman, using the last of the savings she'd kept hidden from her husband during his gambling escapades. She told me, "I wanted to live in a more dignified neighborhood, not the favela, but as an older, single woman whose husband had stripped me of almost everything I had, there weren't many other places I could go. Luckily by that time the city allowed you to buy land in the favela, and I wanted something permanent—a piece of land and a house that I could leave for my daughter when I was gone."

Isabella was thrilled that she managed to buy her home and that she had a title to prove it, but in the years that I knew her, she expressed deep anxiety about the legality of the title. "It's my husband's name that is on the title to the house, not mine," she explained, because she had not consented to formally divorce her husband. "That means if I die before he does, he has the right to the house. Vera won't get anything." I asked her if she could go to a lawyer to try to change this, but she rejected my suggestion out of hand: "What lawyer would listen to me? I'm just a poor woman, and here, mainly in Ceará, husbands always do better than wives."

When I returned to Pirambu in the fall of 2000, Isabella's worries had become exacerbated by rumors circulating in the favela about a pedestrian boulevard that was to be built by the city straight through favela land. Isabella said the city of Fortaleza was hoping to attract more tourists by laying a broad, cement, pedestrian boulevard along the oceanfront from near downtown to Pirambu. All of the houses in the path of or near the proposed boulevard were targeted for demolition. Some residents assured me that the government would reimburse people whose homes were in the way with certificates for occupancy in new apartment blocks being built in another part of the favela. But Isabella wasn't as confident: "Who knows when or if we'll even see this certificate. The city makes lots of promises. It's hard to know which they'll keep."

Meanwhile she was growing more and more anxious about the prospects for her daughter. "This generation has no respect for hard work, Jessica," she told me late at night after Vera had gone to bed. "Look at me—I had a decent job in the city. I made a real salary. But Vera? She doesn't like school. And how is she going to find a stable job in this economy? If I could afford to send her to private school, maybe she would do okay, but I don't have the money for that."

In this context, securing the title for her house to pass on to Vera took on added urgency. She told me she had considered hiring a lawyer through one of the community associations in Pirambu to try to get the name on the title changed. "I don't trust the law," she told me, "but I know that I deserve this land, I'm not a squatter. I made good money and have the right to my home, and I want my daughter to have it too." Despite her strong feelings on the subject, she resisted actually going to the legal association to get help, brushing aside my occasional questions about the matter during the course of my stay.

Isabella's concerns about her house, the legality of its title, and the stability of her daughter's future were common themes in our conversations during my return visits to Pirambu in the summers of 2005 and 2007. The city had yet to follow through on the promise to deliver a certificate of occupancy to a new apartment, as far as she knew construction on the new buildings had not even started yet, and her husband had made several phone calls insinuating that he would be more than delighted to take up residence in her home after she passed away. Meanwhile, Vera successfully graduated from high school in the spring of 2007, but she had yet to embark on a "solid path," according to her mother. "She wants to be a massage therapist," Isabella told me, "one of these flexible jobs where you don't work a lot and don't earn a *salário mínimo* [minimum wage]").[5] But this isn't something that will help her maintain a house, give her a living. How will she pay for the kung fu classes she wants to take? For the new shirts I see her wear?" Isabella was by now in quite poor health, unable to walk long distances in the favela or to complete the many household tasks that previously took up her days. Her thoughts seemed to focus almost entirely on the welfare of her daughter and on a rejuvenated relationship with the Catholic Church.

By the time I returned to Pirambu two years later, in the summer of 2007, Isabella had passed away from a severe stroke. While her death was not unexpected, I was surprised to learn that Vera, then twenty-four, was not thrown out of the house by Isabella's husband, as her mother had long anticipated, but was rather living in a two-bedroom apartment provided by the city in exchange for access to the land on which Isabella's house stood. Vera narrated the events of what transpired with dramatic flourish soon after I arrived in the favela. After her mother's death, she explained, she became very nervous about how much longer she could live in her mother's house. Government officials came to visit her within weeks of her mother's passing and explained that although she had the right to the house and the land where she was living, the city had plans to build in that area, and thus she had to move to a new building where the city would furnish her with an apartment.

Vera said she worried every day about Isabella's husband returning and taking the title to the house away from her and going to the city to claim the new apartment for himself. "I was so nervous," she told me. "Every night I dreamt I would be thrown out on the street—or [even worse in her mind] that I would have to go live with Maria José [Vera's biological mother] with all the grandchildren and nieces and nephews. That wouldn't be fair, Jessica! Dona Isabella bought this house for me, she did everything right, acted correctly so that we would have this house in our family."

I asked if she'd requested help from anyone, and she said she'd enlisted everyone she could think of to prepare her for appearing in court, as the city requested, to transfer title of her mother's house to the new apartment building. But in the end it was her boyfriend's mother, Simone, who became her most formidable ally. Simone, whose husband Vera said was "blessed with a stable job as a postman," lived just outside the favela in the slightly less poor neighborhood of Barra do Ceará. She gave Vera a fancy set of clothes to wear for her court appointment and told her how to talk and walk so she would look "respectable."

"I was still so upset, Jessica. I wasn't sure I would be able to find a way to do it. I thought I would just be treated like trash in court or that Isabella's husband would show up," she said. Instead Vera said she and her soon-to-be mother-in-law appeared very early in the morning on the appointed day, and the city official barely looked at them. Vera turned in her title for her mother's house and in exchange was given a new title and the keys to a small apartment about a half mile from the house.

We were sitting in the small living room area of the apartment that Vera shared with her now husband, Paulo, as she narrated the story. Paulo's computer, a wedding present from his mother, took pride of place on the large bureau that took up most of one wall. The couple was expecting their first child in several months, and though neither Vera nor Paulo had found steady employment, her overwhelming concern was about the nursery they were planning and whether the crib her in-laws purchased would fit through the apartment's small doorways.

Isabella's struggle to secure a house for her daughter highlights the historical achievements of residents living in Fortaleza's peripheral communities as well as the moral frameworks residents use to interpret their sense of belonging to the city. Isabella came to Fortaleza as a self-described hardworking and resourceful young woman who was able to find a steady job in the city. Her description of those days demonstrates that she believed, albeit tentatively, in the possibility of social mobility and incorporation into modern urban life but also that she attributed these accomplishments to her own morally upright behavior as well as to state-sponsored programs designed to address structural inequalities. Her comments about her job were shaded with paternalism as she attributed her happiness at that time to her good boss, but she also remarked on her stable salary and the accompanying health and retirement benefits. She attributed her ability to purchase a home to both her moral character—her ability to save money and survive her husband, whose dissolute behavior she contrasted unfavorably with her own—as well as to the legalization of buying land in the favela.

Isabella clearly benefited from the legacy of the generation of migrants who first settled in Fortaleza and claimed their rights to the city. Although she did not participate in the political protests of the 1940s and 1950s, one can see how the legal achievements of those decades, such as gaining legal title to land in Pirambu, shaped her beliefs in the possibilities offered by her hard work and education in the city. These beliefs are expressed as subjective experience in statements like "I'm not a squatter" and "I have the right to this land." The strong sense of entitlement, to belonging in the city, was even expressed by Vera in her comments about what is fair and that she knew the land was hers; she only had to find a way to "make it right."

But Isabella's and Vera's stories are also inflected with many of the tensions associated with forms of neoliberal economic development that arose in Fortaleza in the mid-1980s. Isabella's concern for her daughter's future was not just the fussing of an overprotective mother; rather it reflected real conditions and uncertainty about a labor market that had moved away from the stable, fixed-income jobs of the past like the one held by Isabella in the pharmacy and toward high levels of unemployment and the embrace of a flexible culture of labor that demands access to private education and endless education certificates. Though Vera, at her relatively young age, interpreted the decrease in formal employment as an opportunity to try out new kinds of careers such as training as a massage therapist, her mother looked on with evident horror and constantly urged her daughter to find more stable sources of employment. And Isabella was quite aware of and vocally incensed by seeing that, as is so often the case in neoliberal economies, the expansion of consumption patterns in the favela was not matched by an expansion in employment opportunities.

Their stories highlight the perceived weakness of the state to secure residents' civil rights. Despite Isabella's and Vera's persistent conviction that the house and land legally belonged to them, they, like the vast majority of poor Brazilians, exhibited almost no trust in the law itself. Isabella refused to talk to a legal association in the favela that might have helped her sort out the question of title because she was "just an old woman" and not someone the law would take seriously. Vera spoke repeatedly about her fears that city officials would take away her title to the land or give it to Isabella's husband. She worried about being "treated like trash" in the courtroom and was insistent that it was help from her mother-in-law-to-be in dressing her up and coaching her so she would not appear to be "from the favela" that secured her title to the new apartment building. These strong expressions demonstrate that for poor residents of Fortaleza the attempt to secure their rights is still a frustrating and often shame-inducing experience and one that prevents citizens like Isabella and Vera from viewing the courts as an arena of redress. Such experiences thereby further undermined the potential for favela residents to exercise their legal rights, including their newly won right to health care.

Conversations in the Plaza

As I described earlier, some of my most astute informants were young women I got to know well throughout the course of extended and repeated fieldwork visits to Pirambu. Among the many advantages of knowing this circle of friends over the years was not only that I witnessed their transition into adulthood and in many cases the fruition of long-held aspirations but also that I saw how their interpretations of their standing in Pirambu and in the city changed over time. A particular conversation stands out to me in this regard, as it illustrates a new subject position charted by young adults in the favela in response to both the possibilities and inequalities embedded in the city's adoption of neoliberal economic policies.

One evening in the summer of 2005 I went with one of the young women, Adriana, to an undergraduate class she was taking on social science methods. For several years Adriana had been working toward a bachelor's degree in international business at the Faculdade Ateneu, one of a growing number of small, for-profit colleges that had opened up in Fortaleza since the early 2000s. The colleges, whose entrance exams were much less onerous than the dreaded *vestibular* that determines entrance to the country's public federal university system, were becoming increasingly popular among Pirambu's younger residents because the colleges receive federal funding in exchange for providing scholarships to low-income students (Araujo 2012).

Adriana, along with two close friends, gained entrance to the college in 2003 and was steadily taking classes at night while continuing to work during the day at a manufacturing company. The value of the education at such colleges was occasionally debated in Fortaleza's newspapers: Weren't the classes too big? Where had the teachers been trained? And very infrequently the question was raised as to why the government was supporting private-public educational partnerships rather than increasing access to Fortaleza's public federal university. But for Adriana, as for all of the women in her circle of friends, the chance to attend college at all was considered an extraordinary opportunity and one that was not even a remote possibility when they graduated from high school just five years earlier. Obtaining a college degree was the clearest sign that they had surpassed their parents' generation in achievements, and it was the first step in the often-recited list of aspirations: a degree, a car, and a house of one's own.

As we ambled out into the night after the hour-long class, Adriana commented that it must have been pretty boring for me, the teacher going on and on like that and not even on an interesting topic. She much preferred her computer class, in which she was learning how to use some of the programs they had on the computers at her work. The class we attended together was full—forty people in a small classroom—and most of the students were texting or otherwise involved with their phones as the teacher lectured. Adriana claimed that the teacher didn't mind: "She gives us all A's anyway. She just wants to get paid."

As we talked we walked to a plaza across the street from the college and met up with two other women from Pirambu, Francine and Sofia, both of whom were working toward degrees at the same college. We bought some french fries from a nearby street vendor and sat down to continue our unhurried conversation. Shortly thereafter, a woman approached our group, looking pitiful and asking for money. Francine, by far the quietest and gentlest of the group, shooed her away with one hand and then turned back to us and explained, "You can't help these people. They'll just want to buy pizza, and you know they all have rice and beans at home," referring to the ubiquitous and cheap Northeastern meal. There was a pause in our conversation around the table, and Francine continued, turning now to Adriana and saying, "This is *cara de favela*, this begging. It's what gives Pirambu a bad name. All you do, if you give in to this, is enable their wants, nothing more. They will never learn, never get it into their heads that they must go and do things for themselves."

Adriana and Sofia were nodding their heads in agreement, and Sofia turned to me and said, "These people are just squatters. They haven't learned how to look after themselves. It's just like my brothers—so undignified!" Sofia, the youngest of eighteen children, had two older brothers who still lived in her parents' house and, she said, did nothing all day long but drink and make a nuisance of themselves.

"It's disgusting," Francine said. "There are women in Pirambu who don't want anything better for themselves or their children. All they want to do is to reproduce and sit around their house. What kind of life is that?"

Adriana agreed and began to speak about her sister who was sixteen and just had her second child: "We all tried to help her, we paid to take her to a private clinic to get birth control, offered to watch her daughter while she finished high school, but she wouldn't listen. She just sits around the house all day and doesn't want to expand her horizons at all."

And here Francine cut in to ask, "Why would you want this for yourself or your children? The only reason to have kids is to give them a better life than you had."

At this point I asked the women what percentage of people in Pirambu had this attitude they were describing and how many people were more like them, trying to get an education and better their lives. Francine was the first to respond to this, saying, "It's really just a minority, Jessica, that want to do better. Most people are *super contente* [very content]. They have this *mentalidade do interior* [rural, uneducated mentality]. You know, everything's okay, they don't want to work too hard. But it's a sad life they have, really."

Sofia added here, "You need so much more to succeed now, not just primary or secondary school—you need to finish high school and to go to university." Adriana chimed in, "You're right! And look, even this won't guarantee you a good job."

Here Adriana began to narrate a harrowing story about her recent brush with unemployment. For nearly four years she had worked as a secretary at a company that sold scaffolding materials. She described the boss as one of the few "bons patrões" she had worked for and as someone who really took an interest in her career aspirations. The year before, her boss told her about a slightly higher-level position in another company and sent her to interview for it. The job had many perks, and Adriana described them all in vivid detail: she would earn more than at her previous job; she would receive two free sessions of computer training; and she would only work from nine to five Monday through Friday, with no work on Saturdays. Although working more than forty hours a week was technically illegal in Brazil, almost all low-wage jobs required at least a half-day's work on Saturday. Finding a job that was only Monday through Friday was considered the holy grail by everyone I knew the entire time of my fieldwork. Adriana said, "It would have been amazing, and with the extra money I earned I could have paid someone to come in to help take care of my mother on the weekends." Adriana's mother suffered from severe depression and anxiety and rarely left the house. As the unmarried, oldest daughter in the family, most of her mother's caregiving fell on Adriana's shoulders, a situation that caused her particular bitterness on Friday and Saturday evenings when she wanted to go out dancing or to dinner with her friends.

Adriana was offered the job shortly after she interviewed for it and quit her other job in short order. Then, just days before she was supposed to start work at the company, the new boss called her and told her the company was downsizing and her position was no longer available. She described her outrage at his attitude during that conversation: "He treated me just like dirt, like he couldn't even be bothered to say he was sorry. As though I hadn't quit this other job already and didn't have my entire family depending on me!"

"Well, what did you do? Did you speak with anyone about this?" I asked.

"I did the only thing I could do," Adriana replied. "I had to go back to my old boss and beg for my position back. Luckily, he's a good boss, very kind, and he took me back." And here she turned to me to finish out the story: "This is what we know how to do best here in Pirambu—you always have to work hard, and you have to chase down your success."

The Moral Discourse of a New Generation

The group of young women with whom I had this conversation as well as other, similar conversations represented a small but not insignificant elite cohort in Pirambu who had both profoundly benefited from the accomplishments of their parents' generation and far exceeded their parents' economic and academic expectations. They came of age in the favela with access to running water, consistent electricity, reliable public transportation, local schools of questionable quality but with open admission, countless community associations, and perhaps most significantly, middle-class yearnings and aspirations.

The three women I spoke with that night lived at home, and the divide in their households between themselves and their parents was stark. Sofia lived above the rest of her family in a single, large room that had an indoor toilet and shower, still somewhat unusual in Pirambu, a large refrigerator and stove, and wall-to-wall, glossy, new tile. She paid for all of the renovations herself from money she saved by working as a massage therapist on one of Fortaleza's many tourist beaches. Meanwhile, her parents and her two much-older sisters lived on the first floor of the house in three cramped rooms, and a varying number of older brothers slept in hammocks in the house's exterior courtyard. Her parents' portion of the house still bore vestiges of their former life in the rural interior of Ceará. They kept an old wooden stove on the patio, refused to exchange the outdoor bucket shower and ground toilet for more modern amenities, and adhered to a solid diet of rice and beans. As in almost all of the households where I spent time, there was a generational tension over the propriety of the girls' ascent into the upper strata of Pirambu's class structure and their embrace of middle-class values and aspirations. Sofia's father discouraged her from finishing high school and was actively campaigning against her pursuit of a college degree.

But in addition to this generational divide I also observed a more rigid class structure emerging in Pirambu. In prior decades the opportunities and aspirations within the community were relatively similar and tended to center on communal goals, while now individual growth and betterment appeared to be the focus of many of the younger residents I knew in Pirambu. As the conversation I related above makes clear, the projects carried with them a moral discourse that justified why some in the favela succeeded while others still had what was perceived as a backward mentality.

Francine's harsh comments about Pirambu's poorest residents sounded almost shockingly like the diatribes I heard from Fortaleza's middle- and upper-class citizens about the whole of the favela. Francine and her friends conveyed frustration with what they perceived in the very poor as a sense of entitlement, expectation of perpetual help, and reluctance and inability to take command of their lives. And the young women extended their critique beyond just some abstract marginal group but also to their own siblings. It was striking that the women did not urge poorer residents to political protest, as they might have done in decades past. Rather, they perceived that the civil and political rights for which prior generations had fought already existed, and they were incensed precisely because some people in the favela seemed to refuse to take advantage of them.

The new subject position emerging in the favela exemplified by the three young women's views of marginality highlights how forms of neoliberal economic governance that have led, on the one hand, to public-private partnerships like the one undertaken by the college the women attended can also produce shifts in moral attitudes toward valorizing individual choice, self-improvement, and picking oneself up by one's bootstraps (Burchell 1996). What is striking is that in less than a generation, explanations for success or failure in the favela have transformed from being attributed primarily to the state's attentions or lack thereof to the hard work and initiative of individuals.

Furthermore, I rarely heard the young adults of Adriana's generation comment on the extent to which the state's earlier contributions to life in the favela—in its provision of utilities, transportation, and primary and secondary education—created the conditions for more far-reaching aspirations. Rather, many young adults in Pirambu, and particularly those who were gaining skills that might enable them to leave the favela behind, measured their success by how many of the opportunities afforded by the increasingly privatized and market-driven economy they could incorporate into their lives. In this context, new kinds of employment opportunities, such as Sofia's job as a freelance masseuse, were much more highly valued despite their instability than, for example, a six-days-a-week, minimum-wage job at Lojas Americanas, the Brazilian version of Target, where several of the girls had worked.

But other parts of the conversation I have described above make clear that reliance on oneself alone is risky business in Fortaleza's emerging neoliberal economy. Adriana's brush with unemployment when the company suddenly downsized showed the fragility of new economic opportunities and the magnitude of what she stood to lose had she not had a boss whom she could ask for her job back. At the time of our conversation, Adriana was the primary wage earner in her household. Her mother was entirely dependent on Adriana's income, and her younger sister and her sister's children depended on Adriana for food and schooling costs. Her father contributed to the household income when he could, but like many men in the favela, he had started another entire family with a new girlfriend and provided for them first. In traditional family structures in the favela, men often support additional families and women become the de facto economic heads of households; these patterns have not changed as rapidly as economic and social opportunities have. Thus young women in the favela may experience far greater opportunities than their mothers did, but because they are often still placed in positions of family responsibility, the younger women put family members in addition to themselves at greater risk by taking advantage of the opportunities.

Moreover, as we saw in Vera's and Isabella's struggles for secure housing, Adriana likewise did not perceive the law as an arena of justice that could be used to exercise her civil rights. I asked Adriana several times if she could have gone to a lawyer when the new job she was promised vanished before she began it. The answer was always the same: "Of course not!" And then she elaborated, "They never would have listened to me, and if I had gone to the law, I wouldn't have gotten my old job back for sure." Thus she was forced to rely on the tried and true method of the favela—the paternalistic favor of a former boss. Although she expressed outrage at her situation, the lack of a principle of legality was totally normalized. Residents of Pirambu, even the most financially stable among them, simply do not expect the state to effectively defend equality, liberty, or dignity in their public and private lives.

Residents of poor and marginalized communities throughout Brazil experience a disjuncture between having fought for and won political rights such as voting in free and open elections and socioeconomic rights including health care while on the other hand not being able to rely on state institutions such as the court system to respect or defend individual rights. This is a well-recognized paradox that reflects new forms of social injustice and inequality (Caldeira and Holston 1999). In this chapter I have provided a historical accounting of the disjuncture by describing the origins and ongoing development of the community of Pirambu and its residents' expectations. As we saw, starting in the 1940s and 1950s residents began to express their social needs and aspirations as the rights of citizenship. Remarkably, through social mobilization and political protest they achieved a broad spectrum of services and legal recognition from the city of Fortaleza before the start of the military dictatorship.

The 1988 constitution made the achievements of favela residents throughout the country highly visible with the special attention it gave to the social rights of women, children, and minorities and its inclusion of new civil rights such as health care. Despite these gains, Fortaleza's and all of Brazil's simultaneous embrace of neoliberal economic forms of governance as well as deeply entrenched patterns of clientelism and paternalism ensures that residents of contemporary Pirambu confront a conflicting mixture of structures of power and meaning as they shape their futures and negotiate their sense of belonging in the city of Fortaleza.

CHAPTER TWO

A History of Welfare and the Poor in Ceará

With the adoption of Brazil's 1988 constitution, universal and equitable access to health care became the guiding principle of the new health care system, the Sistema Único de Saúde. To implement this system, however, its supporters in Ceará had to navigate an already entrenched two-tiered health care structure with many private medical clinics, hospitals, and physicians as well as public medical facilities, community health centers, and state-employed health care providers. One of my goals in this chapter is to describe the historical emergence of the two-tiered health care system in Ceará and its particular, multifaceted character. What could account for a system in which small, public health clinics (*postos de saúde*) dotted the landscape of even the poorest communities in the city and residents went regularly for care and assistance without remarking on the practice?[1] How did preventive medicine become an underlying goal of Brazilian health care and embedded in the way the state delivered care? And finally, how had private medical clinics, which Pirambu's younger residents were beginning to seek out, survived after successive decades of strong federal support for public health services?[2]

In providing this history, I focus on the relationship between what might most broadly be termed "welfare" and Ceará's poorest residents and more particularly on the ideologies that underlay successive eras of health-related welfare assistance.[3] During the colonial era the poor relied almost exclusively on Christian charity for intermittent medical care. Under the republic (1890–1930), addressing the population's health came to be seen as a political necessity throughout Brazil, and federal intervention into matters of health was increasingly supported. Though still largely inaccessible to the majority of Ceará's residents, medical services expanded rapidly throughout the state during this period as the idea of improving the public's health took root and preventive medicine was adopted as a legitimate model of care.

With the Vargas administration's linkage of health care benefits to certain categories of labor, residents of Fortaleza's low-income neighborhoods began to agitate for specific health care services and greater access to medical care. As I describe later in this chapter, the social history of health care in Fortaleza poses a challenge to prior scholarly accounts of the relationship between health care agencies and the poor. Those accounts tend to emphasize the control that dominant classes have exercised over lower classes through medicine and focus almost exclusively on the ways that health policies and practices regulate and discipline people's everyday experiences (Comaroff 1994, Farquhar 1994, Hirschfield 2008, Scheper-Hughes 1992). Historical evidence from Fortaleza suggests that low-income residents were more directly involved in the actual expansion of health care services than has been reported in other geographic areas. And in a theme that is recapitulated throughout the book, in this chapter I describe the involvement of the poor in the expansion of specific medical services and draw attention to how individuals become active subjects in the creation of health care ideologies.

Charitable and Military Initiatives in Ceará's Colonial Era

The history of welfare in what is now known as Ceará began in the late 1600s with the construction of a single medical clinic in the region, known as a *hospício*. *Hospícios*, established by the Jesuits throughout Brazil during their tenure, were a mixture of convent, college, and hospital (Barbosa 1994, 28). As with other colonial medical institutions of the New World, they took in the sick and provided food and assistance to invalids and the poor (Brodwin 1996, 26). The institutions are thus best understood as not exclusively or even primarily addressing medical concerns but rather as providing Christian charity in a range of contexts including sickness, old age, and destitution.

A second formal medical institution, the Hospital Real Militar, was constructed in 1769 as part of a military compound in what is now Fortaleza nearly ten years after the expulsion of the Jesuits from Brazil and the abandonment of many of their *hospícios*. Maria Nobre, a historian of colonial medicine in Ceará, notes that the hospital was built with a grant from the Lisbon government in response to epidemics that continually swept the area and to the ongoing needs of soldiers stationed in the compound (1978, 97). Although the hospital served both settlers and local Indians who had been enslaved by the early villagers, its main role was to provide medical care for soldiers to ensure continued colonial dominance.

In letters back and forth between crown and colony, prominent settlers consistently stressed the need for better medical services and for treatment for soldiers who were attacked in raids by indigenous populations in the area. They complained that the local infirmaries were miserable and often produced disease instead of quelling it (Nobre 1978, 104). In 1798 the governor of Lisbon finally ordered that additional doctors and a surgeon be sent to the Hospital Real Militar, but the soldiers' productivity remained paramount; population health was yet neither a concern nor a goal of the early medical institutions.

The other prominent type of medical asylum of the era was the charitable Santa Casa de Misericórdia (Holy House of Mercy), a Catholic institution which, like the Jesuit *hospício*, served the sick and the destitute.[4] Though they were found widely in other parts of Brazil during the colonial period, Ceará did not see the implementation of a Santa Casa until 1861. Upon its completion the institution became known for introducing modern surgical procedures to the region as well as hosting European doctors who would teach classes and practice medicine for months at a time (Barbosa 1994). Brought into the SUS in the late 1980s, the Santa Casa de Misericórdia remains a functioning hospital and is a beautifully kept building in downtown Fortaleza, but its reputation among residents of Pirambu is ineluctably tied to its humble origins; like the public graveyards in which they did not want to be buried, residents associated the Santa Casa with marginalization and disgrace.

The Emergence of Public Health in the Old Republic

Up through the nineteenth century, medical services for the vast majority of Ceará's residents, to the extent that they were available at all, came in the form of charitable assistance. Exceptions to this included the use of technical expertise in mass quarantines and public education campaigns during the epidemics and droughts that periodically swept the state. But it was not until the late nineteenth and early twentieth century that the general health of Ceará's population became a political priority and a policy objective.[5] During the first several decades of the twentieth century, public health reforms and services in Ceará, as in Brazil more generally, expanded rapidly and were characterized by significant support from the federal government and an overt commitment to social change.

By the late nineteenth century, health conditions in all of Brazil's major cities were deteriorating. Waves of infectious diseases such as yellow fever and smallpox reached the port city of Salvador and then quickly radiated north to Recife, Natal, and Fortaleza and south to Rio de Janeiro and Santos (Castro Santos 1987). Worried about the impact of disease-ridden ports on the country's immigration policies and trade interests, Brazil's first president, Prudente de Morais (1884–1898), created a federal department of public health in 1897.[6] Additional federal health policy was developed under the administration of President Rodrigues Alves (1902–1906), including granting the federal government direct responsibility for regulating sanitary conditions in all of the country's port cities and supporting a massive vaccination campaign against yellow fever and bubonic plague in Rio de Janeiro (Castro Santos 1987, 102–106).

In 1916 doctors Belisário Pena and Atur Neiva from the Instituto Oswaldo Cruz, a newly created research center on infectious diseases, published a medical survey of the Northeastern *sertões* (the back country away from the Atlantic coast in Northeastern Brazil) that described in detail devastating conditions of poverty and illness, including the widespread presence of conditions such as hookworm disease, trachoma, yellow fever, tuberculosis, and schistosomiasis.[7] In the study, 70 percent of the rural population was found to have hookworms, 40 percent was afflicted with malaria, and Chagas disease was found in 15 percent (ibid., 130).

The physicians' report helped to galvanize public support for increased federal intervention and spending on public health, but it also introduced a sharply critical and explicitly political voice into the national discourse on health. Rather than relying on commonly accepted explanations for poverty and disease such as environmental conditions, the authors argued that it was the subordination of power to large landowners, the feudal living conditions, and the lack of government aid that were the real causes of Northeasterners' impoverishment and misery.

The overtly political arguments were analogous to those made by a small, new group of medical doctors and sanitation experts, the *sanitaristas*, who focused on urban sanitation in the late 1910s and early 1920s. Led by several medical doctors who had specialized in public health at

Johns Hopkins University in Baltimore, they argued for a new model of public health to create health centers responsible for preventive actions such as mother and child hygiene, immunization, and sanitation education (Stralen 1996). The *sanitaristas* were successful in securing resources from the federal government. For example, in 1929 the federal government funded courses at the medical school in São Paulo to prepare doctors for executive positions in public health administration. By linking health problems to social and economic issues and taking on roles in key government posts, the *sanitaristas* opened up space for understanding health care reform as an instrument of social change (Castro Santos 1987, Estorel 1999, Magalhães 1980, Stralen 1996).[8]

By 1918 public support for federal intervention in health services had built to the point that the Brazilian Congress passed an act to create a Ministério da Saúde (Health Ministry). The act transferred all services regarding health from other government agencies to the new body and stipulated that it would be in charge of promoting sanitation in ports, cities, and the interior of the country. The act thus concentrated responsibility for public health services in the hands of the central government and reduced the role of state governments, which had been in control of health services since the 1889 advent of the republic. President Epitácio Pessoa (1919–1922), an ardent supporter of health care reform, issued a new sanitary code in 1919 that was passed by the Congress the same year. The code gave stronger powers to the federal public health service, and by 1922 almost one hundred *postos sanitários*, basic primary care units, had been opened in the neediest areas of the rural interior of Brazil (Castro Santos 1987). By the end of Pessoa's term, public health campaigns had become a major goal of national politics, and rural health services had become firmly centralized under federal authority.[9]

Among the Northeastern states, Ceará was relatively slow to benefit from the federalization of health services. Its backland regions were not among those surveyed for the Pena-Neiva report, and its capital city, Fortaleza, was dwarfed in importance by Salvador and Recife, the centers of the Northeast's sugar economy at the time. Nonetheless, the establishment of select federal health programs in Ceará helped to organize and expand medical services throughout the state and supported a model of health care that emphasized preventive rather than curative care delivered at community clinics. Remnants of this model persist in Fortaleza to this day.

The most influential federal program to reach Ceará during the Old

Republic was the Serviço de Profilaxia Rural (Rural Preventive Health Service). President Venceslau Brás (1914–1918) created the service in 1918 as an official quininization program for rural populations afflicted by malaria. Federal taxes on alcohol, pharmaceutical products, and licensed gambling were used to fund the program, which quickly expanded to include the prevention of Chagas disease and hookworm disease. The service opened an office in Fortaleza in 1920 under the direction of Dr. Antônio Gavião Gonzaga, a local leader in public health. The historian José Barbosa notes that the office served as a place where local doctors would meet to exchange ideas about the burgeoning field of public health and to discuss the implementation of modern medical practices throughout the state (1994, 93).

One of the first actions of the Serviço de Profilaxia Rural in Ceará was to create health clinics in the interior of the state, in Sobral in 1922 and Juazeiro do Norte in 1924, and to open a primary health care facility, the Centro de Saúde de Fortaleza, in 1933. Modeled on institutions that had grown rapidly in the United States and Europe after World War I, *centros de saúde* began to appear in Brazil in 1925 under the direction of Dr. Geraldo de Paula-Souza, the country's sanitation director.[10] Paula-Souza called attention to widespread problems with Brazil's sanitation services and argued for the creation of permanent health centers that would contain a public health department and provide sanitary and health education. He won the support of the federal government, and centers were built in major cities throughout Brazil; they prioritized the preventive health needs of the surrounding communities, developed response plans for major epidemics, and coordinated health education campaigns (Castro Santos 1987, 220–222). Although doctors initially protested the implementation of these services, by the mid-1930s *centros de saúde* could be found throughout Brazil.[11]

Governor of Ceará Carneiro de Mendonça noted in 1933 that the Centro de Saúde de Fortaleza represented a point of pride for the people of the state capital because it successfully centralized a disparate set of public health services in Ceará and was the first center in the Northeast to provide hygiene and nutrition instruction at the prenatal, preschool, and secondary school levels (Mota 1997). The passionate support of governors for health services like Fortaleza's Centro de Saúde was crucial in states like Ceará, where state politicians were required to vie for federal funding for such services.

Throughout the 1930s health services in Ceará continued to be centralized through a series of reforms known collectively as the Reforma

Pelon, elaborated by the *sanitarista* Amílcar Barca de Pelon. The reform movement brought attention from the Departamento Nacional de Saúde (National Health Department) to Ceará, and in 1934 the state was divided into five *distritos sanitários* (public health districts), with Fortaleza serving as the district headquarters in its new Centro de Saúde. In 1936 Fortaleza Mayor Raimundo Alencar Araripe formalized the city's public health services and signed a law creating a city health department as well as a public sanitation department (Mota 1997). In 1939 the municipal health department was restructured, and Fortaleza's Centro de Saúde was integrated into the state Departamento de Saúde Pública (Public Health Department).

Thus in a span of only two decades, federal support for public health in Ceará and the backing of committed state and local politicians helped to create health departments, expand public medical facilities, and centralize the state and municipal public health services (Mota 1997). The acceptance of federal intervention in health policy in the early twentieth century, and particularly the explicit embrace of a model of preventive medical care that emphasized the political dimension of health, set the tone for the way health care was thought about and practiced in Fortaleza for the remainder of the century. The commitment to preventive care in the early twentieth century can be linked to the continued, widespread acceptance and use of community clinics found throughout Pirambu and other low-income communities from the 1950s through the 1990s and 2000s. More broadly, the persistent though sometimes minority view of understanding health as a sociopolitical problem rather than merely a technical one laid a foundation for the introduction of the Sistema Único de Saúde in the late 1980s and into the 1990s (Coelho 2013). These trends were also compatible with an earlier model of health care, developed under Getúlio Vargas, that made it a welfare benefit for certain categories of laborers. It was during his administration of 1930–1945 that Pirambu's residents began to play an active role in the creation and expansion of medical services.

Health Care as Welfare

In a moment of extreme hyperbole in 1937, Brazilian journalist José Soares Maciel Filho wrote, "The Brazilian worker, by virtue of the system of social legislation adopted in Brazil, enjoys job security, paid vacations, and free health care, has access to financial assistance in case of illness, is protected in case of work mishap, and is guaranteed care-free leisure in his old age by his government pension" (in Levine 1981, 17). He was describing Getúlio Vargas's new social welfare program, Previdência Social. Though few Brazilian workers would ever enjoy the parade of benefits extolled by Soares, the introduction of the program denotes a shift in the political landscape that followed the onset of Vargas's administration. Under the Vargas program of national reconstruction, state bureaucracy was expanded, the government's role in shaping economic development was broadened, and a new relation was fostered between the state and the urban workforce. The introduction of the modern welfare state in Brazil, by which I mean a state that actively promotes and protects the economic and social well-being of its population, offered a fundamentally different way of providing health assistance to the poor, one that reconceptualized medical services as an individual benefit to be given in exchange for labor rather than as a form of charity or population health control.

Of all the programs inaugurated during the early years of Vargas's presidency, among them an expanded set of labor laws and a new labor court system, it was Previdência Social—social security—and the health care services created to fulfill its mandate that would have the most direct impact on residents of Pirambu. The first step taken by the Vargas government to develop a social security program was to expand the old system of the Caixas de Aposentadoria e Pensões (CAPs, Retirement and Pensions Funds) in 1930–1931 to include public service workers, miners, and dock and maritime workers. Medical assistance would be offered in conjunction with the scheme only until additional legislation for health services was created, and funding for all forms of medical assistance was limited to 8 percent of the annual federal budget (Stralen 1996, 42). Despite the restrictions, the idea that insurance schemes like CAPs should include medical care was gaining ground.

The link between retirement and health care was strengthened in 1933 by the federal government's initiation of the Institutos de Aposentadoria e Pensões (IAPs, Retirement and Pension Institutes), which organized workers' insurance by occupational category rather than by individual companies. Each institute defined its own set of benefits and was regulated according to its own internal policies. Most IAPs, facing direct competition from other institutes, were unable to resist their members' demands for medical coverage. Medical services were sometimes delivered from the provider's own facilities; more often, however, the services were contracted out to private providers including fee-based doctors, clinics, and hospitals. The contracts prompted rapid growth of the private medical sector and set the stage for the development of a two-tiered, public and private health care system.

In May 1945, months before he was removed from office, Vargas expanded Previdência Social by creating the Instituto de Serviços Sociais do Brasil (Institute of Social Services of Brazil). It was in line with an international movement after World War II to embrace the idea of providing equal rights to basic security and welfare regardless of class or status position; the agency was meant to provide cradle-to-grave protection for all Brazilians, encompassing retirement and survivor benefits, extensive medical care, and a full range of social services such as sick pay and disability support. While the law supporting Vargas's institute was rescinded the year he left office, the share of the Previdência Social budget allocated to medical care nonetheless increased from 5.4 percent in 1946 to 19.3 percent in 1960 (Stralen 1996, 60).

The number of direct contributors to Previdência Social doubled as a result of the new system, going from close to two million in 1940 to more than four million in 1960 (ibid., 72). As with the old system, the quantity and quality of services delivered by the institutes varied widely, largely because wages determined the revenue a given IAP had to spend on health services. The IAP Industrial (IAPI, the IAP of industrial workers) had less money to spend on health care than other IAPs because industrial workers earned substantially less than other employment sectors such as banking, medicine, and law.

By 1954, many of the approximately twenty institutes that had been established were delivering services through their own health agencies and had begun to invest substantially in building outpatient clinics and hospitals. The number of hospitals created by the IAPs rose from a total of five in 1948 to twenty-eight in 1966. Nonetheless, their networks were still insufficient to provide medical services to all of those who had insurance, particularly those who lived outside of major cities (Stralen 1996, 80). Thus, nearly all of the institutes continued to contract services out to private providers, thereby again greatly increasing the private medical sector at the expense of the public sector and further solidifying the two-tiered public and private medical system I found in Fortaleza at the end of the twentieth century.

From the time he was reelected in 1950 until his death in 1954, Vargas continued to develop Previdência Social, primarily by adding to the list of occupations that were covered by the system. In spite of the expansion of medical assistance, access to medical care in Ceará continued to be quite limited, and the great majority of workers, including rural laborers, domestic servants, street vendors, and thousands of others in the informal urban economy, did not benefit from the growth of Previdência Social, tied as it was to participation in the formal labor market. As in previous eras when the poor had been dependent upon charitable assistance or public health schemes such as vaccination campaigns, formalized health services remained largely inaccessible.

Political Activism and Health Care Services in Pirambu

While the early benefits of social insurance may not have reached most residents starting to build their homes on the edges of Fortaleza, the idea that members of society could be guaranteed the right to certain benefits because of their participation in the labor market was nonetheless compelling. As welfare benefits were introduced and grew under President Vargas, residents of low-income neighborhoods around Fortaleza began to clamor for the extension of resources and services to their own communities.

The startling headline of an article from 1947 read, "Queremos Comida e Remedios! clamamos moradores do bairro do Pirambu" (We want food and medicine! residents of Pirambu shouted). Describing a demonstration against the conditions of misery in which Pirambu's residents lived, the article detailed their appeals for adequate medicine and a health clinic in the neighborhood (*O Democrata*, September 27, 1947). Their appeals were explicitly political in nature and framed in the language of citizens' rights and government's responsibilities. The same article notes that one of the slogans in the demonstration was "O governo devia era cuidar do povo" (What the government should do is take care of the people), and the demonstrators criticized the government for not paying attention to the suffering of ordinary people. An article in *O Democrata* a year later, on September 9, 1948, carries the headline "O povo do Pirambu luta por posto médico, chafariz e calçamento" (People of Pirambu fight for a medical clinic, a [public] well, and street paving). The article emphasizes the demands made by Pirambu's residents to the city's politicians and notes that they blamed the community's impoverished conditions on Fortaleza's mayor.

A review of Fortaleza's three major papers from 1940 through the early 1960s reveals that one of the most frequent demands by Pirambu's residents was for more medical facilities in the community. A small health clinic was established in 1949, but it was quickly overwhelmed, and residents began clamoring for additional clinics. In 1950 a women's organization in Pirambu, the União Feminina, met with members of Fortaleza's city council to request the installation of an additional medical clinic (*O Democrata*, September 5, 1950). The organization's representatives reportedly told the council members that residents of Pirambu, "não suportando a miséria que assola seu barrio, está decidida a lutar pela melhoria de suas condições de vida" (not tolerating the misery that devastates their neighborhood, have decided to fight for improvements to their living conditions) (*O Democrata*, October 28, 1950). The president of the city council promised to study the case and seek funds for the construction of a clinic.

It was ten years later, however, when Pirambu finally received a major sum of money from the state government to finance a medical clinic and to make other improvements in their neighborhood. In 1960, following years of demonstrations by community residents, the governor of Ceará Parsifal Barroso agreed to give five million cruzeiros to Pirambu. The money was to meet specific needs identified by residents in the areas of education, clean water, and medical facilities (*Gazeta de Notícias*, May 24, 1960). In 1961 the state government granted an even larger sum, again for the construction of clinics and schools (*Gazeta de Notícias*, August 5, 1961).

That year six clinics were opened throughout Fortaleza in low-income neighborhoods specifically for serving populations that the city health department had not yet reached. Following a municipal ordinance enacted more than twelve years earlier, in 1948, by Fortaleza Mayor Acrísio Moreira da Rocha, the health services office and these clinics were free of charge for all residents (Mota 1997, 43). The clinics provided basic medical care and, in keeping with historical health policies, emphasized hygiene as the main strategy to combat illness and promote health. Although the clinics did not provide extensive medical resources for low-income residents, they did offer tangible evidence of the potential benefits of mobilizing for rights.

In the early 1960s, city officials viewed improvements in the area of health care as essential to the development of Pirambu. A set of plans outlined by the city government in 1960 for developing Pirambu included recommendations for the state health department to establish a health education center and a maternity center in the neighborhood (*Gazeta de Notícias*, May 19, 1960). An article in the *Gazeta* the day before identified eight key areas to improve Pirambu, four of which were medically related, including dentistry, maternal and infant protection, health education, and clinical medicine. By the early 1960s, then, residents and city officials alike understood health care as a salient political resource that denoted a certain kind of belonging to the city of Fortaleza.

Anthropologist James Holston (2008) has cautioned against too favorable an interpretation of Vargas's reforms for urban workers. He argues that Vargas's innovations did not constitute a new model of citizenship, as is often supposed, but rather a modernization that perpetuated the nineteenth-century paradigm of "differentiated citizenship," which sharply restricted the number of workers who were actually given access to social rights. What appears to me important about the Fortaleza case, however, is that despite the small number of favela residents who may have actually attained the social rights introduced during the Vargas era, their gains appear to have encouraged other members of the urban poor to seek such rights for themselves.

Newspaper records provide dramatic evidence that as early as the mid-1940s there were movements among low-income communities like Pirambu to secure social rights such as health care and other domestic services for themselves. Even more noteworthy is that the demands were articulated in a specifically political language—the government should take care of the people—thus signifying their belief that they should have "the right to have rights" (Arendt 2004, Holston 2008) and drawing attention to the state's inherent responsibility to the world they shared. In so doing, residents were at least partially successful in extending the resources of the emerging health care sector to the poor. The intensity and success of these movements suggest that although Vargas's benefit programs may have been intended to discourage autonomous organizations on behalf of the urban poor, at least in Fortaleza, their introduction effectively broadened working-class mobilization.

Health Care and Community Activism during the Military Regime

On March 31, 1964, President João Goulart was deposed by the Brazilian military, and General Humberto de Alencar Castelo Branco was installed in his place. During the two decades of military dictatorship that followed, Brazil underwent a process of complex sociopolitical changes that transformed the country into a modern industrial power with social welfare programs while simultaneously deepening socioeconomic inequalities within and between regions. This kind of paradoxical effect occurred in Fortaleza, where even though private and public health care institutions and services proliferated largely through the growth of Previdência Social, they continued to exclude the urban poor from medical coverage and care.

The persistent exclusion of poorest urban populations from health care coverage was the direct result of social policy, for although the categories of workers to whom welfare benefits were allocated continued to expand—allowing, for example, domestic workers to obtain health care benefits in 1972—these benefits remained tied to employment rather than to one's status as a citizen of Brazil. Because benefits remained tied to the wages earned in a particular sector, jobs that offered higher wages also offered more benefits and services to their employees than others; disparities arose such as bank employees being guaranteed full health care benefits, while most industrial workers were not (Stralen 1996). This kind of differentiation supports Holston's observation that in Brazil, one could technically be considered a citizen while still being caught in a system of status differences that prevented him or her from enacting citizenship to acquire important services and protections. One of the most important changes brought about by the SUS was the guarantee that health care benefits would be linked at the outset to citizenship rather than to employment.

The inequities in health care coverage did not go totally unnoticed by a military regime in need of political legitimization, but attempts at ameliorating the problem often ended up simply exacerbating it. In 1974 the newly created Ministério de Previdência e Assistência Social (Ministry of Social Security and Assistance) launched the Plano de Pronta-Ação (Plan of Immediate Action) to make health care more broadly accessible to the beneficiaries of Previdência Social by allowing them to use their allotted benefits to purchase services from any provider, public or private. Following this decision came a rapid expansion in the number of private providers of ambulatory and hospital care. However, data from this period suggest that lower-income groups were actually harmed by the expansion, as private hospitals tended to deny access to patients who were unable to pay fees for better accommodations or were not fully covered by health insurance (Stralen 1996, 119). Poorer patients were sent to crowded public hospitals or to *postos de atendimento médico* (medical clinics) run by the Instituto Nacional de Previdência Social (INPS, National Institute of Social Security) that were springing up in lower-income neighborhoods throughout Brazil's major cities including Fortaleza. It is already possible to see here the expansion of the two-tiered health care system so visible by the time I arrived in Pirambu in 1998 to conduct fieldwork, in which patients of different socioeconomic backgrounds were purposefully assigned to different medical centers and institutions and there received starkly different standards of care.

Low-cost preventive health programs were another idea supported by various bureaucrats in the military regime as a way to address the inequities in Brazil's health care system. In 1976 the Programa de Interiorizacão de Acões de Saúde e Saneamento (PIASS, Program for Ruralization of Health and Sanitation Actions) was created. PIASS was initiated in Northeast Brazil to provide low-cost preventive and basic curative services to rural communities through a large public network of health centers and clinics using locally trained health care workers. Although the program was forced to shut down several years later due to lack of federal funding, the unofficial motto "simple medicine for simple people" used by PIASS officials would became a model for highly acclaimed low-cost health care programs (Stralen 1996, 125). The programs garnered praise from the international development community but reinforced a split in medical care that was already lamented by Fortaleza's working class: low-tech, prevention-oriented medical care for the poor and high-technology care for all who could afford it.

The dominant narrative for health care during the military dictatorship was decidedly that of government-sponsored growth of health care services, both private and public, and the accompanying expansion of Previdência Social. As I have stressed, the extension of benefits to a broader range of workers rarely benefited the urban or rural poor and ultimately served to consolidate the two-tiered medical system that was firmly in place when I arrived in Fortaleza in 1998. This is not, however, the only available narrative to explain the development and expansion of biomedical care in Fortaleza during that time.[12] For, as in the Vargas era, working-class movements eventually began to play a role in defining the health care needs of and securing medical services for their neighborhoods.

During the 1970s, public awareness of Brazil's social and health inequalities grew rapidly as the "economic miracle" that marked the military regime's early years began to falter and the process of *abertura* (opening) encouraged protest against the regime's social policies (Escorel 1999).[13] In Fortaleza in 1979, taxi drivers, bus drivers, and train operators went on strike for higher pay. For some political commentators, the strike symbolized a return to protests that had been dormant in the city during the dictatorship, and helped to restart movements by the urban poor for better health care and other social services (Farias 1997). Among the most important accomplishments during this time was the formation of the ABCs, the Associacões de Bairros e Conselhos (Associations of Neighborhoods and Councils). The associations were formed in low-income communities throughout Fortaleza and other cities throughout Brazil to assess the needs of community members and articulate them to city representatives. Although initially the Fortaleza associations were isolated from one another, by the early 1980s they had formed an umbrella organization and appointed representatives who entered into dialogue with city officials about health care and other issues (Alencar 1992).

What was important about the associations with regard to the history of health services for the poor was their ability to define the specific health needs of their communities and then to persuade city officials to address them. One of their earliest projects was to inform city officials about the poor conditions of maternal and infant health in the favelas. In response to these reports, in 1975 the city launched the Instituto Nacional de Alimentação e Nutrição (INAM, National Institute of Food and Nutrition) and the Programa de Nutrição em Saúde (PNS, Program of Nutrition in Health); the institute and its program provided nutrition and health advice for pregnant women and infants who lived below the poverty line in Fortaleza (Braga 1991, Mock 1997). Several years later the city joined the National Milk Program of the federal Secretaria Especial de Habitação e Ação Comunitária in cooperation with community associations to provide free milk to children up to the age of seven who were living in low-income communities. One of the unique features of this program—and something that would presage a guiding principle of the SUS—was that it was community associations rather than city health officials who selected the families that were to receive the free milk (Braga 1991, 84).

During the gradual transition from a military dictatorship to democracy, which reached completion in 1989 with the first direct presidential election in twenty-nine years, the impact of community organizing in Fortaleza notably increased. Starting in 1986 the federal government and the state of Ceará as a whole began to encourage the systematic participation of laypeople in governmental programs. This marked a fundamental shift in government policy and was seen as a great victory by social activists in Fortaleza (Braga 1991). The progressive incorporation of popular movements into city politics coincided with the 1985 mayoral election of Maria Luiza Fontenele of the PT, an outspoken advocate for the city's poor. During the mayoral terms of Lúcio Alcantara (1977–1981), César Neto (1981–1984), and José Maria de Barros Pinho (1984–1985), popular organizations did not achieve consistent access to city government officials. With the election of Fontenele, progressive social organizations throughout the city became institutionalized and developed long-term ties with city and even state bureaucracies.

The organizations that emerged at this time, such as the Federação de Bairros e Favelas (FBF, Federation of Neighborhoods and Favelas) successfully maintained a dialogue with city officials and pushed for further reforms in the area of health care. Marches organized by the FBF prompted Fortaleza's Secretaria do Trabalho (Labor Department) to construct preschools and health clinics in low-income areas and to support the state-funded Programa de Suplementação Alimentar (Food Supplementation Program) in its continuing development (Braga 1991, 92). In 1987 the Programa de Creches Comunitárias (Community Preschool Program) was expanded, and community leaders were invited to participate in the design of new educational programs. And in 1988 the União das Comunidades da Grande Fortaleza (Union of the Communities of Greater Fortaleza) was formed as an umbrella organization to put representatives from all low-income communities in contact with city officials, including medical care planning commissions, and to initiate the building of a series of health and outpatient clinics in Fortaleza's poorer neighborhoods.

Medical Pluralism in Ceará

By the end of the military dictatorship, the field of medicine in the state of Ceará was centralized, highly stratified, and deeply medicalized and professionalized. It was a mixture of public and private institutions, public health and social welfare services, and preventive and curative medical care. Throughout this chapter I have tried to stress the multiplicity of local and national, community and state, and public and private forces that produced this curiously mixed field of medical care and practice.

During the colonial era, medical services for the majority of Ceará's residents, to the extent that they were available at all, came in the guise of charitable assistance. With the birth of the republic and the consequent consolidation of Brazil as a nation-state, national health services slowly became accepted as a political responsibility. Several federal health programs reached Ceará including the Serviço de Profilaxia Rural, which was responsible for the creation of several health units in the interior of the state, and a primary health care clinic in Fortaleza, the Posto de Saúde Central.

The spread of medical services in Ceará during the republic was directly linked to their transformation into political, professional, and bureaucratic entities. Residents in rural areas but particularly residents in the city of Fortaleza were increasingly likely to encounter medical institutions and practices in their daily lives because of the services' proliferation in the state as a whole. In the southern cities of Rio de Janeiro and São Paulo, health was coming to be understood as an abstract good that was in some measure the duty of the state to provide; by the early twentieth century at least some of the policies and institutions necessary to support this concept had taken root in Ceará.

The Vargas administration strengthened the nascent understanding of health as a duty of the state by creating social welfare programs that offered health care as a benefit of employment. The administrative centralization required to implement these programs increased the power of political elites in Ceará and allowed them to substantially augment medical resources and services, particularly in Fortaleza. Using federal funds designed to improve public health services, the local *sanitarista* Amílcar Pelon advocated centralization of health policies and divided the state into five districts, each responsible for monitoring and serving a specific population.

In many ways the military regime's response to health care was an intensification of trends begun under the Vargas regime. The number of medical institutions and providers in Fortaleza increased dramatically due to the rapid expansion of Previdência Social; but health care benefits remained tied to employment, health care services continued to be centralized, and the private medical-industrial sector that began to emerge during the Vargas regimes was strengthened during military rule through the support of state intervention and policies that favored private medical practice. Increasingly, the health care system was acquiring a two-tiered character with an essentially privately funded system offering high-quality health care for privileged groups of the upper and some middle classes contrasting with a publicly funded, impoverished, lower-level system for the masses of rural and urban poor.

Although the spread of medical care under the Vargas and military regimes primarily served the middle and upper classes, Fortaleza's low-income residents played a crucial role in the extension of at least some medical resources and services to their communities. What was striking about these movements was their expression of a political consciousness that saw health care not as the benefit of employment that Vargas and the military regime wanted to suggest but rather as something that should be guaranteed by virtue of citizenship as proposed in the Sistema Único da Saúde. Specifically, protests during the Vargas and military eras were not cries for extending employment benefits to an ever-growing list of workers but were calls on behalf of specific communities for services to which residents felt entitled as residents of Fortaleza.

The protests pose a challenge to scholars who attribute municipal health reforms primarily to federal and state bureaucrats, state and national lawmakers, and rural and urban oligarchs (Barbosa 1994; Castro Santos 1987, 338), and they point to another set of social actors in the spread of biomedicine. While not discounting the profound importance of government intervention into health politics or the extent to which the urban and rural poor were systematically excluded from successive eras of health care reform, Fortaleza's history demonstrates that we cannot neglect the potential of popular movements born out of assertions of belonging to the city to expand the reach of health services and medical practice into their communities.

In the past two decades social movements regarding health care have slowly been transformed in Pirambu. Voluntary associations focused on health care issues have closed as politicians direct residents' attention toward participating in the democratic health councils described in the next chapter, while residents mobilize around domestic projects, family health, and in the case of some younger residents of Pirambu, around the consumption of private health care.

CHAPTER THREE

Democratizing Health Care: Health Councils in Pirambu

We have to radicalize democracy; that's exactly what is missing from the Partido dos Trabalhadores [Workers Party] at the national level. Popular participation will be something absolutely new for Fortaleza.
—LUIZIANNE DE OLIVEIRA LINS, MAYOR OF FORTALEZA, JANUARY 2005

In the years that followed the military dictatorship, political and civic leaders began an intense public discussion of Brazil's health care needs and policies. The policies adopted during this period responded to an ongoing crisis in the country's social security system as well as to the intensifying social and political demands for health care reform. In 1986, at the landmark 8ᵃ Conferência Nacional de Saúde (Eighth National Health Conference), a unified and decentralized health care system was outlined that was eventually to become the Sistema Único de Saúde. The SUS imposed extensive changes on the health care sector, among them the transfer of health services and financial resources from federal to state governments, as well as more fundamental shifts such as the redefinition of health care as an obligation of the government and a right of citizenship. All of the reforms proposed at the conference and later enshrined in the 1988 constitution have received considerable political, popular, and scholarly attention but perhaps none so much as those defining the participation of ordinary citizens in the prioritization and delivery of their own health care (Bógus 1998; Coelho 2007, 2013; Cornwall 2007, 2008; Cornwall, Cordeiro, and Delgado 2006; Galvanezzi 2004).

The 1988 Brazilian constitution stipulated that the new health care system be governed according to democratic criteria and include the participation of civil society in its decision-making processes. In order to enact these principles, *conselhos de saúde* (health councils) were to be created at the federal, state, and municipal levels to help plan and supervise health care actions. The councils were to be composed of service providers, government officials, and—most provocatively—local residents, who were to make up a full 50 percent of council membership.

The inclusion of a local voice in health care planning is not, on its own, a new or necessarily radical idea. In her work on the politics of primary care in Costa Rica, medical anthropologist Lynn Morgan notes that international development agencies have been using the concept of citizen participation as a kind of health development panacea since the 1970s (1993, 45). In Brazil, the *movimento sanitário*, a health care reform movement started in the early twentieth century by public health specialists, envisioned community engagement in the provision of services as a key component of health care reform. And, as we have seen, residents of Pirambu repeatedly struggled to have their voices heard in the effort to widen access to health and health resources. But the formal participation by Brazilian citizens in health-related decision making was not seriously considered by the federal government until it was presented as a way to regulate the transfer of funding and health services from the federal to the state level, a process that was itself at the heart of the health care reform agenda (Stralen 1996).

Almost since their inception, Brazilian health councils at the municipal and neighborhood levels have been the subjects of careful ethnographic and sociological research. Authors have evaluated the councils' potential to offer new spaces of democratic deliberation and participatory government (Cornwall 2007). Some have studied their effectiveness at promoting citizen participation and offered important suggestions about how the councils might include the most disadvantaged members of society and enable them to play a meaningful role in defining public policy (Coelho 2007, Martins et al. 2008).

Here I offer a different kind of account of the *conselhos de saúde*, one written primarily from the perspective of residents living in Pirambu, only some of whom were even aware of the existence of the new health councils, let alone had ever participated in them. I give a detailed account of one of several meetings I attended in Pirambu led by a local doctor to generate interest and eventually participants in the municipal-level health council meetings held in Fortaleza. My analysis of the meeting highlights the tensions that surfaced between the residents' and the doctor's definitions of key conceptual categories such as health and participation. The eventual dissolution of the meetings and the inability to find anyone interested in attending the higher-level health council meetings was interpreted by the doctor as a failure to generate sufficient community interest in matters of health and a sign that community participation in health care at the neighborhood level was an unattainable goal. Then I provide an alternative interpretation of the perceived failure by offering examples of the local idioms and practices through which Pirambu's residents redefined health and participation as a kind of collective responsibility.

Conselhos de Saúde, an Introduction

On one of my first days doing fieldwork in Pirambu someone mentioned there was a health care clinic just up the hill from where I was living. The clinic, it turned out, was a small cinderblock house nearly indistinguishable from its neighbors. It was run entirely by the good grace and indomitable will of Dona Mariata, an older woman who was trained as a midwife and offered her services and the supplies mostly donated by visiting foreigners to residents in the immediate vicinity. By her own testimony, she had delivered hundreds of babies over the years, but at the time we met she primarily treated people with minor ailments and referred them if necessary to the municipal clinic several hundred feet up the road.

I visited Dona Mariata often during my first stint of fieldwork in 1998–1999 as well as on all of my return visits over the next decade, soliciting her information and opinion on, among other subjects, health and health care reform in the favela. But it wasn't until toward the end of one visit in July 2005 that the topic of the *conselhos de saúde* came up.

The lack of conversation in Pirambu about the health councils during the early years of my fieldwork was perhaps not surprising, given the local political context. Fortaleza's Conselho Municipal de Saúde (Municipal Health Council) was established in 1995 as regulations were implemented throughout the state requiring the establishment of councils in order to gain access to federal health monies. Fortaleza's mayor at the time, Antônio Cambraia, as well as his immediate successor, Juraci Vieira de Magalhães, belonged to the generally centrist political party the Partido do Movimento Democrático Brasileiro (PMDB, Brazilian Democratic Movement Party) and did not have a strong interest in popular participation as a form of governance. Reports from the period suggest that from 1995 to 2005 the council functioned in name but was widely perceived as being a rubber stamp for the decisions of elected officials. In January 2005, Luizianne Lins of the left-leaning PT was elected mayor, and with her close connections to social movements and a commitment to popular participation in municipal government, she almost immediately turned her attention to health care reform. Following her election, political rhetoric about popular participation increased substantially, and by the time I arrived to conduct follow-up fieldwork in the summer of 2005, newspaper articles and televised news reports were repeating the same, ubiquitous message of getting the people into the government. Lins was quoted in an interview as saying, "We are planning to build in all of Fortaleza's neighborhoods popular organizations that will enable everyone to discuss problems with city hall and with the mayor" (Lins 2005).

The expansion of local governance was to include the creation of local health councils in the city's poorest neighborhoods where residents could express their interest in and opinions about health matters; eventually several of the residents would be elected to attend the larger, more formal Municipal Health Council meetings held in downtown Fortaleza. When I began fieldwork in the summer of 2005, I read various articles about this idea in the local papers, but several months in I had yet to hear anyone in Pirambu discuss the creation of the local health councils or comment on their imminent arrival.

On one particular day, however, late in the humid month of July 2005, I noticed a thick bulletin stapled to Dona Mariata's door announcing the inaugural meeting of a local health council in Pirambu that was to take place several days later. I turned to Mariata and with some excitement asked if she knew anything about the meeting and whether she was planning to go. She eyed me warily and said, "Esses conselhos de saúde não funcionam muito, não, Jessica" (These health councils don't function very well, Jessica). Then she asked me to help her drag the crate of aspirin inside that had been sitting on the doorstep of the clinic.

Defining "Health" and "Participation" in Pirambu

Despite Dona Mariata's stern retort, I ended up attending three health council meetings during the summer of 2005, after which the idea of sustaining a local health council in Pirambu was abandoned altogether. The first of these meetings took place in August, before a new *posto de saúde* (health clinic) was to be built in Pirambu. The objectives for the meeting were to draw up a list of health care priorities for the clinic and to promote awareness of the Municipal Health Council operating in Fortaleza. The meeting was publicized in the days leading up to it through fliers distributed throughout the neighborhood and over the loudspeaker of an advertising bus that rumbled up and down the favela's alleyways.

A young, male doctor who worked for a public hospital in Fortaleza ran the meeting, which took place in a local community center primarily used by a grassroots legal group dedicated to providing free legal advice to residents of the favela. As the meeting began, twenty to twenty-five community residents filled the room, most of whom were women. The doctor started the meeting by explaining that the reason he was there was because one of the mandates of the Sistema Único de Saúde was to include local residents in decisions about what kind of health care they would like to see in their communities. He went on to inform the audience that within the next year a new clinic would be built in the neighborhood and that in order to ensure that it met the community's medical needs, city health officials needed the residents' help in defining what those needs were.

"So," the doctor continued, "why don't we start by naming some of the most common health problems in the area. What kinds of health issues bother you most?" The room fell silent for several moments while the participants looked at one another, whispered to their neighbors, and fell silent again. Finally, the residents began to speak. "We wait in line too long," one woman called out. "Safety," said another. The doctor asked her to expand on this: "What do you mean by safety?" She responded, "You know, we can't go anywhere in this neighborhood at night—how am I supposed to feel safe walking alone, or worse, with a sick family member to the clinic? And then waiting there? How can I wait there, just waiting to be robbed?"

Another woman chimed in, "Yes, we always feel unsafe here. It's terrible to expect that we'll wait outside for someone in the clinic to see us." The doctor jumped in at this point and, sounding surprised, asked, "Do you feel unsafe during the daytime too?" Residents agreed that they felt most unsafe at night. "But," one woman said, "night is when people most often have emergencies."

"What about other problems?" asked the doctor. "What kind of ailments do you have the most trouble with, the flu? Colds? Is asthma a problem here?" Residents responded by naming a host of problems that troubled them and their families. The final resulting list included, prominently, waiting in line, safety, lack of medicines, and unavailability of ambulances as well as rats and hunger.

The doctor responded that he would be happy to address these general problems but that toward the end of the meeting they should probably discuss the specific health problems they were experiencing as well. "Let's begin with the safety problem first, as many of you seem very concerned about this issue" he proposed. "I understand that you feel frightened and that older people in particular are reluctant to leave their homes. But what can we do about this?" One woman said she didn't know and added, "Just yesterday there was an assault in the supermarket up the street—at 2 p.m., in broad daylight."

"You know what you need to do?" asked the doctor. "You should form community groups that take turns acting as night-watch people. You could also walk in pairs to the health center and that way reduce your chances of being involved in an assault. And you could call the local community associations and ask for better street lighting." There was silence in the room. Some residents nodded their heads, while others looked unsure. The doctor continued, "The whole neighborhood has to work together to solve the safety problem. It's not going to go away on its own. You are much more powerful as a group, and you should act together."

Then the doctor added that in the meantime, residents could offer to walk with older people to the health center and that doctors themselves could begin to visit older people in their homes so they wouldn't even have to go to the center. This received a murmur of approval. "In fact," the doctor went on, "with the new health center we're planning to put here, public safety can increase simultaneously with the installation of the new center. We might install a doorman to guard the health center at night, and maybe we'll have enough money to put in street lights around the center."

"Can we go on?" he asked. "Let's talk about item number two, the lack of medicines. Why is this a problem?"

One of the women in the audience responded, "When we go to the health clinics, there's nothing there. The medicines we need are always gone. And then we either have to pay for them ourselves or we're sent to another health unit to get them, and they may not have them either." Another woman seconded this complaint: "It's true, I almost never get the medicine I need from the health clinic near my house. I thought the new health care system, the SUS, was going to change this. I thought it meant we would get the medications we need."

The doctor didn't answer this directly. Instead he asked the residents why they thought there was a shortage of medications. Very quickly people responded. "Because people steal them from the center, and then they sell them!" one said. "Yes," said another, "I've seen this. I know that people sell the medicines. Sometimes they take them to use, just like drugs. But most of the time they just sell them to make money." A woman said, "Drugs are such a problem in this neighborhood, we see them all the time." The man sitting next to her agreed, saying, "It's true, it's getting to be as bad as the south. Even my uncle said he thinks drugs are a problem here, and he's from Rio."

Amid all the responses the doctor stepped in and said, "You know what you can do about this? You can tell people. If you see bad behavior, people stealing or using drugs, you should report it. You should denounce your neighbors. This is your responsibility, as a good neighbor, as a citizen of Fortaleza. You can create a good, safe neighborhood to live in, but only if you report bad behavior and if you tell officials—only if you denounce your neighbor."

Residents said they were afraid to speak out against certain neighbors for fear of retaliation. The doctor responded that wasn't a problem because they could do it anonymously. "The most important thing," he said, "is that you begin to speak out, to imagine the kind of community you want, the kind of neighbors you want, and that you put this vision into action."

He went on to admit that the lack of medications in the health clinics could be because the community leaders who ran them were giving medications to people outside of the area the clinic was supposed to serve. He continued, "The health post that we're going to build here is going to be just for you, just for the people who live in this area. This is the only way we can make the system work. Otherwise, too many people will try to take advantage of the clinic's services."

He then explained, "We're going to work hard to make a list of all of the houses in the area and check people off as they come in. Then we'll only give medicines to the people on this list. You should also know that every family will have a file where all the health notes will be kept about everything that has happened healthwise to that family. This will allow us to keep track of what medicine is needed for which person, and it will prevent us from giving medication to people who don't really need it."

The next problem on the list was the lack of ambulances. The doctor began to address this issue when a woman interrupted him to ask, "What about the rats? Rats are a much bigger problem in the neighborhood. Everyone I know has them." Another said, "It's just disgusting. How are we supposed to be healthy—with these rats?" The doctor replied, "You're right. This is something that needs to be addressed. You can't go on living with rats and expect to be healthy. But this also is an area where you have to help yourselves. You should go to your community leaders and ask them to help you. You also need to be careful about where you put your garbage. The rats come because they smell the garbage that you've left outside your homes. Are you dumping the garbage in the main dump?"

"It's too far away," a woman replied, "and we can't always get there. It would be much easier if we could leave our garbage in a place that was more convenient." The doctor asked, "Why don't you organize a group of people to take turns bringing the garbage to the main dump? That way no one will have to do it all the time. This is another area where you should educate your neighbors, about how to handle garbage, and report those who are simply dumping garbage in the streets to leaders in your neighborhoods. You see, there are many things that can be done to take care of the rat issue, but you cannot act alone. You have to act together."

The final topic left on the list was hunger. "We don't have much time left, but what did you want to say about the issue of hunger?" asked the doctor. A woman explained, "I don't understand how I'm supposed to be well if I'm hungry all the time." One said she was very worried about her children not getting the nutrition they needed. And a third woman responded, "You see this all the time here, these children who are living on practically nothing, trying to fill themselves up on sacks of chips. This is no way to eat. I don't see—how does the government expect us to be healthy when these are the conditions we live in?"

The doctor replied that they didn't have enough time to finish the conversation but that at the next meeting they would begin where they'd left off. "I also want you to think about real health problems that you or your neighbors have that this health clinic could address," he said. "This will help us draw up a list of priority medicines and ensure that the clinic is equipped with the appropriate technology." He wrapped up the meeting by reasserting his main message: "You need to act together to get the help you want. Most of all you should imagine the kind of community you want to live in and develop the grassroots organizations, the community power, and the will to bring that kind of community into being."

With this pronouncement the meeting broke up, and people began to wander out of the room. As I was leaving, I overheard an elderly woman say to her friend, "This reminds me of the old days, don't you think? When we used to march to city hall to demand health care."

Assembling Definitions of Health

The health councils mandated by the SUS were designed for the explicit purpose of allowing local communities to prioritize their own health care needs. However, a closer examination of the health council meeting I've just described reveals that the community residents and the doctor leading the meeting were using conflicting definitions of "health," which made achieving even a relatively simple goal such as prioritizing health care needs more difficult. The doctor leading the health council meeting in Pirambu consistently appealed to a definition of health that could be described in terms of illness and disease categories and the services and resources needed to treat them. Even his first question to the group—"What are the most common health problems in the community?"—assumed that there was already a shared understanding of what constitutes a health problem.

Despite the doctor's willingness to listen to residents' broad responses and to offer possible solutions, throughout the meeting he stubbornly returned to a definition of health that fell within the parameters of biomedicine. "Let's discuss these things," said the doctor after the initial list was drawn up, "but let's get back to the health problems at some point in the meeting." And he finished the meeting by again asking participants to focus on problems the clinic could address and medications and technologies it would need.

Residents, on the other hand, consistently articulated a much less conventional definition of health. In response to the doctor's first question, about common health problems, they brought up a broad array of topics not confined strictly to disease categories. Their responses about waiting in line, hunger, rats, and safety all center on systemic problems within the favela that neither health councils nor the SUS is necessarily equipped to resolve.

Even examples that explicitly referenced normative definitions of health, such as the concern about the lack of medications quickly spiraled into a conversation about people stealing medication either to sell in the drug market or for their own consumption. That topic in turn led to a conversation about the issue of drugs in the favela in general. From the residents' point of view, these issues were intimately connected to health itself.

Scholars have argued for years that in order for basic health care initiatives to succeed, health care workers must acknowledge that poverty itself is often the principal cause of disease (Farmer 2003; Holmes 2013; Mechanic 1999; Van der Geest, Speckman, and Streefland 1990). In fact, the idea that improving people's health must be linked to the resolution of basic issues such as safety, adequate nutrition, and decent housing has had many precedents in the history of Brazilian health care reform. *Sanitaristas* in the 1920s argued that given the huge social inequalities in Brazil, attempts to improve health conditions could not be restricted to formulating specific health targets but rather had to involve a broad process of social change (Stralen 1996, 241). This concept of health was widely endorsed at the National Health Conference in 1986. Its final report, which directly preceded the formation of the Sistema Único de Saúde, stated, "In its most comprehensive meaning, health is the outcome of the conditions of nutrition, habitation, education, income, environment, work, transport, employment, leisure, access to land and possession of it, and access to health services" (ibid.).

Nor are doctors and other health care professionals who work in Fortaleza unaware of the myriad of challenges favela residents face in their daily lives and the obstacles these pose to becoming healthy. Following the meeting, I asked the doctor how he thought it had gone, and he replied, "It was basically as I thought it would be—this is a high-risk area because of all the drugs and a lot of violence. We see this all the time because the conditions are so poor for people to live in. But the main problem here is that people must be educated in order to learn how to accept the kind of health care they're being provided with."

"What do you mean by this?" I asked.

"Well," the doctor said, "they have to be educated in the arena of preventive care and not just come in demanding medicine for this or that problem—this is what they generally want, a quick fix. There are so many things they don't understand about how our medical system works. They don't understand, for example, that there are certain days you come for particular problems and kinds of care—such as, you must come for a prenatal visit on Wednesdays, not just any day of the week."

Here, he threw up his hands in exasperation. "So, you have to teach them that there are certain categories of illness, kinds of care they can receive on certain days. Otherwise it adds to our work load enormously."

Although progressive definitions of health, ones that link the possibility of health to the necessity for social change, have been present throughout the long history of Brazilian health care reform, what this conversation with the doctor demonstrates is how difficult the ideology is to sustain in practice. Doctors, confronted on the ground with spectacular levels of poverty and daily hardships, often resort to advocating for narrower definitions of health problems that they can redress with appropriate biomedical services and resources. In order to do this successfully, however, they first have to reeducate residents about what the term "health" encompasses and what they can reasonably expect from a health center.

The doctor's attempts during the meeting to steer the conversation back to specific health categories, as well as his explanation of carefully tracking families' medical histories and only offering medications to those residents living within the health clinic's designated area, were all efforts to demonstrate how good health might be achieved by understanding and following normative biomedical practices. His more explicit statements to me after the meeting reflect both his recognition of the challenges favela dwellers face and his perception that residents' health is dependent on their adjusting their expectations of what medical care actually is and becoming educated about how to access it appropriately. But that process is itself political; it calls for a strictly biomedical understanding of the body and medical practice in which the vital characteristics of residents and communities become the subject of interrogation and control (Rose 2007). Residents' responses in and outside of the meeting show their discomfort with this model and point to the discontinuities between it and local understandings of health and community.

Participate! Participate! Participate!

I go back to the quiet conversation I overheard as residents were filing out of the initial health council meeting. "This reminds me of the old days," a woman was saying to her friend, "when we used to march to city hall to demand health care." At the two subsequent meetings the older residents in attendance continued to comment on the similarity these sessions had to earlier protest movements led by community activists to secure health care and additional rights and services. "We've always been loud—a big mess for the city!" remarked one woman of the community of Pirambu.

In some respects it did not surprise me that the health council meeting would remind older residents of the social protest movements they carried out during the 1950s and 1960s. In both situations, residents of Pirambu were articulating desires for social rights and services and focusing on the question of how to improve their community. There were also, however, important differences between these two forms of social practice.

During the 1950s and early 1960s, residents' energies were directed toward securing a guarantee from the municipality of Fortaleza for the extension and fulfillment of a spectrum of social services. The self-organized political protests seen in the decades before the military dictatorship and emerging again in the 1970s were part of a broader struggle against a pervasive culture of authoritarianism in which rights were conceived as favors or gifts from those in power. In demonstrating for the right to adequate medical facilities, favela residents were struggling to persuade government officials that they were not the idle, marginal people of popular description but rather decent, working-class citizens worthy of bearing rights (Dagnino 2005, Holston 2008). What the older residents of Pirambu with whom I spoke at the meetings remembered most often about these politically charged periods was the necessity to continually remind Fortaleza's leaders of the favela's existence. One older gentleman who spoke with me following the last of the health council meetings remarked about the earlier eras of protest: "The strength came from us—our people here in the neighborhood. If they [the people in city hall] had the right to drink a glass of water from a faucet, we had to show them that we had it too."

Residents of Pirambu had experienced extensive changes to their community in the decades leading up to the summer of 2005, when the health council meetings began. Neighborhoods in Pirambu now enjoyed a number of the services for which residents had lobbied years earlier, including running water, electricity, public transport to the city center, and a sprinkling of health clinics. Perhaps most dramatically, the 1988 constitution extended political and civil rights to the Brazilian populace including not just access but the constitutional right to health care. All of these changes signified potentially profound gains for the city of Fortaleza's poorest residents.

But the health council meetings I attended highlighted an accompanying shift in how and on what terms residents engaged with public officials. The doctor leading the meetings had not, for example, encouraged residents to demonstrate against the city government as they had in earlier eras, nor had he suggested that they lobby their local council members for additional social services or demand that the newly elected mayor fulfill her many promises. Rather, the doctor urged residents to invest their energies in a wide variety of community betterment projects, such as forming a crime-watch group, accompanying elders on clinic visits, and lobbying city officials for street lights.

These discussions and others I heard like them at follow-up health council meetings reveal a general pattern I observed in the favela of leaders external to the community urging residents to participate and improve their neighborhoods by working on their own behalf. The concept of community participation as a supplement or in some cases a replacement for state services is similar to descriptions other scholars have given of the repurposing of social movements in new democracies throughout Latin America (Dagnino 2007, Paley 2001).

Suggestions of directing energy away from demands for public services and toward their private fulfillment were received with ambivalence by many of the residents participating in the meetings. Several complained after the meeting that too much of the responsibility for improving conditions in their community was being put on their shoulders. A woman commented, "There is a lot of community involvement here in Pirambu. I don't want to have to organize yet another community group to get better lighting. This is something that the mayor said would happen. They've been telling us for months that they're going to improve the lighting here." Other comments I heard between the meetings included "Why should I come to these meetings? They just tell me to work more than I already do" and "I thought they were coming to us because they had the solutions."

Their remarks echo those that scholars have documented in response to community health initiatives around the world (Stone 1986, Ugalde 1985). Van der Geest, Speckman, and Streefland sum up the problem succinctly: "People do not want self-reliance if it means they will be left to fend for themselves" (1990, 1030). But in the context of Pirambu, residents' remarks also reflect a pattern of frustration I observed repeatedly in the favela at the accelerating erosion of boundaries between public and private responsibilities that was ironically concurrent with the expansion of selected rights for lower-income Brazilians.

In addition to urging favela residents to find ways to participate in and work together for the good of their community, the doctor also overtly encouraged residents to identify bad neighbors and to report unlawful behavior. Using the rubric of personal responsibility, the doctor reminded them that it was their responsibility as good neighbors and citizens of Fortaleza to help make their neighborhood a safe place to live. Part of this project of good-neighborliness, the doctor asserted, was defining where the boundaries of residents' neighborhoods lay. He mentioned several times the need to produce a list of all the households in the neighborhood that would be served by the one particular health clinic that would be created.

As with the push for greater community involvement, residents were ambivalent about taking on an overt policing role in the neighborhood and of the idea that a kind of sovereign neighborhood could be established to accomplish this. "Why should I denounce my neighbors?" a woman asked "We know each other here." Another commented, "We can't do anything about the guys on drugs anyway. You need to be stronger—to be part of the police force—to do that." Here, favela residents recognized the fragility of the networks of reciprocity and patronage that defines favela life as well as the essential, fluid, and inclusive boundaries of their neighborhood. Not only are they unlikely to be able to significantly reduce violence in the favela on their own, formally speaking out against neighbors also violates codes of conduct essential for belonging to a dense urban neighborhood that demands a politics of inclusion rather than exclusion.

Recasting the Form of Participation

Enthusiasm for the health council meetings quickly dwindled; by the third meeting there were only a handful of residents in attendance, and the doctor decided not to hold any more. "We had hoped to find someone from Pirambu to go to the Municipal Health Council meetings in Fortaleza," the doctor told me after the last meeting, "but I just don't think there's enough interest in this process." When I asked him why, he offered the following explanation: "*O povo pobreza* [poor people] aren't very sophisticated. They don't think with a long view about how to improve health for their children or their grandchildren. They're thinking about what they can do today—[about] what they need right now."

Residents with whom I spoke about the meetings confirmed the doctor's assertion that their lives were plenty busy just getting through the day: "We just don't have the time, Jessica" was a common answer when I asked them why they didn't want to go to any more meetings. A woman pointed out that as the one responsible for her household of seven, it was unlikely she'd be able to get away and even less likely that she could find someone to send in her place. "Something always comes up in this house," she said. "It's never a good time for me to be running off. And how could I send my husband?"

Residents seemed wary of attending the larger health council meetings outside of Pirambu. "It's just a lot of words," an older man told me. "What would we be doing at one of those big hall meetings downtown, anyway?" As with interpretations advanced by international aid agencies and others advocating community participation in health (Morgan 1993), the doctor interpreted the failure to generate participation in the health council meetings as a reluctance on the part of residents to engage with basic democratic processes and even as a lack of interest in the long-term health of their communities.

While it was true that formal participation in the health council meetings at all levels seemed to have little meaning to residents of Pirambu, my observations over years of fieldwork suggest that they did in fact participate—repeatedly, effectively, and open-heartedly—in matters of health and community, albeit in different terms than those outlined at the council meetings. Residents of Pirambu, and particularly older residents, addressed health matters by participating not at an individual level but at the level of family and community.

Practicing Participation through the Family

While the health council meetings emphasized techniques necessary for the individual management of illness, residents of Pirambu generally do not approach the health care system as individuals but rather as members of families. Visiting a clinic, buying medication, and interpreting diagnoses—these were all mediated by family relations. This tendency can be illustrated in the following examples.

In August 2007 Caterina, the mother of a Pirambu resident I knew well, suffered a series of strokes. She initially was taken to a large public hospital in downtown Fortaleza and, under SUS mandates, was entitled to stay there until she got better or passed away. Caterina's family, however, decided to bring her back home almost immediately. Ana Luisa, one of her daughters, explained to me, "The doctors said she might recover from her stroke there, but we had to take her home. It just wasn't right for her to be lying in the bed without her family. In a private hospital the doctors might have been able to do something, they tell you what's going on, but where she was, they just come in when it's an emergency and they don't tell you anything. We couldn't let her die like that."

They arranged for an uncle who lived in a favela nearer the hospital and could borrow a truck from his employer to transport the old woman back home, and she now lay in a rented hospital-type bed that took up nearly all of the family's cramped living area. Delivery of the bed took several days to arrange and involved calling in a favor from another of Caterina's daughters, Olívia, who worked as an *empregada* (housekeeper) for a wealthy family in one of the fancier neighborhoods of Fortaleza. The family that employed Olívia had a connection at a nursing center and arranged for a bed at a very small fee, which was to be deducted from her monthly paycheck.

While the family expressed great relief at having Caterina back at home, the strain of around-the-clock caregiving was starting to show. Her two eldest daughters moved into the home to care for their mother, dispatching other relatives to take over the daily chores in the sisters' own households. They expressed great reserve about letting certain family members become involved in their mother's caregiving, dismissing a sister who wanted to come from the interior to help because, they said, she had "little knowledge of things." I was told, "She knows how to cook and clean but not how to use these machines the doctor gave us," the intravenous and feeding-tube equipment. Caterina's husband was in frail health as well and was sent to stay with relatives elsewhere in the state for the duration of his wife's illness because he was deemed "too feeble to be of any use around the house" and he "shouldn't have to watch his wife suffer." The younger children in the household were sent to neighbors' homes so they wouldn't be underfoot.

Despite the extensive planning and sacrifices necessary to keep Caterina at home, the family stuck to the regimen, rounding up extended family members and neighbors when the caregivers needed to go back to work or grew tired. "This is not a way to live," one of the sisters confessed to me. "I've been asking God to let her go because it's so difficult for us. But it's important that when she goes it's here at home." When I asked if they would consider taking her back to the public hospital, given that it wouldn't cost them anything, she replied that the public hospitals were for the *pobreza*, the poorest of the poor, and couldn't give her mother a "good death."

Not all residents were as intent on keeping their family members out of the public hospitals; even in these cases, though, the family typically played a strong supporting role. A patriarch of a family I knew well fell ill with a severe case of pneumonia. After trying to call an ambulance for several hours, one of the man's daughters contacted a friend with a car, and the father was transported to a public hospital across town. The man's sons advocated bringing him home soon after he was admitted, but the women in the family, on whose shoulders the caregiving would almost certainly fall, decided it would be easier on his wife if he stayed in the hospital.

Despite the man's placement in the hospital, his daughters immediately created a detailed schedule for who would take the three cross-town buses required to get to the hospital daily and who could sit with him through the night. One of his daughters explained to me, "The hospital isn't nice, Jessica. It's full of people from the *interior*, but at least they let us sit there with him. If we could get him into a private hospital, he would get more attention and not have to be in a big, open room with everyone else, but this is all we can do." Despite doctors' suggestions that the family pick up the medications from the hospital pharmacy, his daughter took all of his prescriptions to a friend who worked at a local pharmacy and would fill them at a discount. Her friend was also sought out to interpret coded medical terms the daughter heard the doctors use in reference to her father.

After several weeks of his hospitalization, one of his daughters had to quit her job in a local dress store to attend to her father. And a young girl who lived several doors down was hired to help with the cooking and cleaning that was piling up at home. When the man passed away almost two months later, the sense of relief in the house was palpable. Immediately an uncle who built coffins was called in, and a place in a private graveyard was negotiated through a client of a granddaughter who had a thriving massage practice.

The social practice of familial reciprocity described in these two examples is not unusual in Northeast Brazil, where extended families and neighbors regularly look after and offer hospitality to one another (Ansell 2007, Scheper-Hughes 1992). But it can be at odds with the rights-based logic of the SUS, which promotes the individual's rather than the family's integration into the health care system. In the examples I shared above, both families used their extensive social ties to secure their own ideas of what constituted good medical care, to locate the appropriate medical resources and information, and to ensure the continued functioning of their households. While they participated in the health care system, they also rejected certain aspects of it, such as the doctors' promise that Caterina's mother would get better if she stayed at the public hospital or the suggestion that the other family leave the older man alone at night. For these residents and particularly for the older residents I knew in Pirambu, the family was the space par excellence where people participated in the health care system.

Practicing Participation through the Community

Despite their resistance to participating in the new, democratic arenas of the SUS, older residents of Pirambu often contributed unremunerated and unrecognized labor to projects that functioned outside of the formal health care system. This form of practice was evident in countless examples I observed throughout my time in Pirambu but was perhaps best exemplified by the work of Dona Mariata, the community resident who maintained the small clinic described earlier. Her personal trajectory as a health care worker as well as the projects she carried out within her neighborhood illustrates ways that some residents of Pirambu strategically use aspects of the formal health care system to advance more personal and local goals.

Dona Mariata was born in 1941 in Missão Velha, a small town at the southern tip of Ceará. She lived in Missão Velha for forty-four years, until 1985, when she moved to Fortaleza with her family to take care of a sick aunt and with the hope of sending three of her daughters to high school.

Dona Mariata herself had only completed elementary school and didn't learn to read until she moved to Fortaleza and took an adult literacy class offered in Pirambu. She also took a class about medicinal plants taught by doctors from the Universidade Federal. She explained,

> All children born in the *interior* know basic things, like how to make *lambedores* [medicinal syrups] from banana, papaya, and sugar. But what I learned in the interior, that was only a small amount of knowledge. What I really know comes from the courses I've taken since moving to Fortaleza. When I arrived in Pirambu in 1985, some doctors from the Universidade Federal were offering courses for mothers in the favela, teaching them how to make certain cures from medicinal plants and confirming ones that we already knew. Dr. Adalberto [one of the doc-

tors teaching the course] was concerned that we were only using drugs, clinical medicine, and wanted us to learn more about how to use our plants.

The classes promoting the formalization of traditional medicine appeared to be precursors to Farmácia Viva's establishment of medicinal gardens and clinics around the city. (Chapter 4 has a detailed description of this program). Dona Mariata spoke about the courses with admiration: "I learned so much about these plants that I didn't know, Jessica. We were introduced to new plants and shown how to make our remedies in a very correct way. Everything I learned in that class and from Dr. Matos [Francisco Abreu Matos, a Farmácia Viva cofounder] I use in the clinic. I love to learn."

Along with the courses she had taken in traditional medicine, Dona Mariata also received training in midwifery and nursing through certificate programs offered sporadically at public health clinics in Fortaleza. As she gained further training, Dona Mariata steadily built up a following of residents in Pirambu, generally women who would come to see her for prenatal care, delivery of their babies, on-the-spot care for mildly sick children, and general medical advice and information. Despite her contributions, Dona Mariata was rarely financially compensated for her work. Sometimes neighbors paid a small fee to see her or offered payments in kind, but more often she simply accepted the charity of friends and family who ensured she was well fed and had other basic necessities.

Although she received little money, Dona Mariata made numerous connections in her years working as a health care specialist in Pirambu with the middle- and upper-middle-class city health officials who occasionally visited the favela to assess health needs and instigate various projects. These connections Dona Mariata put to immediate use in her quest to find better educational opportunities for her children and grandchildren. Over the years I was there, three of Dona Mariata's grandchildren attended private elementary school with the help of a city doctor. She was in the process of negotiating with another city official she knew for her grandson's admittance to a private course to improve one's chances at attending the city's only free public university, and she hoped to be able to get one of her sons-in-law into a private program to train city police officers. Despite her contacts with a relatively broad segment of the health care system's officials and her familiarity with their involvement in health care reform, Dona Mariata's own goals for these connections remained personal: "I want my children and grand-children to have a better life than I did, to maybe one day be able to bring our entire family from the interior to live in the city."

In addition to running her small health clinic, Mariata contributed considerable time to other community improvements. The year I met her, she had just begun a recycling project in which neighborhood children were tasked with collecting empty plastic bottles in the favela streets, washing them, and bundling them for eventual sale in the city. She was particularly proud of this initiative because it addressed what she understood as two of the more serious problems in her community: lack of jobs for the young and the amount of trash that collected in the favela's streets.

When I asked a sampling of friends and local residents to comment on the contributions of Dona Mariata and other local activists to the community, they consistently identified this form of service, local community improvements, as the most important kind of political engagement. Most residents, young and old, had little interest in the citywide or statewide politics surrounding the health care reforms, nor did they believe that the current reforms or the officials who promoted them would necessarily be long-lasting. Community work, by contrast, directly addressed quotidian problems that seemed largely unimproved in the neoliberal era—the need for jobs, for a cleaner living environment, and for better educational opportunities. The doctor leading the health council meeting who urged residents to work together to resolve problems in their community did not recognize that they had, to an impressive degree, already done so and that it was in fact one of the most active forms of civil society in which they engaged as residents of Pirambu and of Fortaleza.

Active Citizenship

The idea of active citizen engagement in the formulation, management, and monitoring of health care policy has been discussed at length in academic and developmental policy literature (Bógus 1998; Coelho 2007, 2013; Cornwall 2007; Jacobi 2000). Less often addressed is how the call for engagement is perceived by people living on the margins of society, where formal democratic processes often remain abstractions.[1] I have argued that particularly older residents of Pirambu tend not to associate health care or community participation with individual rights or formal democratic processes. Nor do they think of their community as divided into carefully delineated zones to which they pledge allegiance. Rather, as we have seen, residents of Pirambu conceptualize fluid neighborhood boundaries and generally participate in the health care system at the level of the family and community structures to gain access to those resources that have the most relevance to their daily lives. This process of tending individual health needs in the context of family and addressing their own community's problems reinforces residents' sense of political community at the local level and is itself a form of democratic practice—and not, in Mayor Lins's words, "an absolutely new one" at that.

CHAPTER FOUR

Prescribing Knowledge: Farmácia Viva and the Rationalization of Traditional Medicine

Many of the programs associated with the Sistema Único de Saúde, such as the health councils discussed in chapter 3, were first elaborated in federal agencies; however, because spending of health care funds was entrusted to the municipalities under the SUS, several locally developed therapeutic programs were used to support the goals of the health care reforms. Farmácia Viva, which was created to teach low-income residents in Fortaleza about the scientifically correct use of traditional medicine,[1] is an excellent example of how local programming became intertwined with state and national health goals.

In 1991 the municipal government of Fortaleza established a public health program called Farmácia Viva (Live Pharmacy) with the aim of "stimulating the practice of phytotherapy,[2] especially in public services, and thus offering an efficient means for the correct utilization of medicinal plants in substitution for traditional household practices and the plethora of industrialized medicines usually offered at exorbitant prices" (Abreu Matos 1998, 23).[3] In conjunction with the Farmácia Viva program, existing health care clinics in various low-income communities of Fortaleza were chosen where local residents could learn scientifically correct usage of traditional medicines and gain free access to medicinal plants and remedies. Scientists at the local university were employed to test medicinal plants for their pharmacological properties and toxicity levels and to provide a list of medicinal plants that would be suitable for the program. Why at this particular historical moment, some six years into the implementation of the Sistema Único de Saúde in the state of Ceará, would the municipal government of Fortaleza, its public health officials, and its university scientists have turned to traditional medicine as a way of improving basic health care services for the city's lower-income residents?

I argue here that if you closely examine the historical origins of the Farmácia Viva program and its component parts, what you find is the promotion of an extremely narrow kind of traditional medicine, one whose form, terminology, and social practices more closely resemble those associated with biomedicine and thus that the program indeed conformed quite closely with the standardization of medical care generally encouraged by the SUS. Public health workers' appeal to validate the use of medicinal plants also reflects their particular imaginations of favela residents as desiring a return to the traditional rural ways of the interior.

Origins

The Farmácia Viva program was first presented to government officials in late 1990 by a group of scientists at the Universidade Federal do Ceará as a way of addressing the health care needs of low-income communities on the edges of Fortaleza's city sprawl. By all accounts, city officials were enthusiastic about the plan and since the program's inception have continued to offer financial and technical support for the project. The ability of the municipal government to support the new program was to a large extent dependent upon crucial changes that had been made in the structure of Fortaleza's health care delivery system following the mandates of the SUS.

The most important of these changes, the shift of allocation of resources from the federal to the municipal level, a process known as municipalization, was well under way in the state of Ceará when the Farmácia Viva program was initially presented as a formal government program in 1991; the city's access to revenues for health expenditures had just been augmented by increasing the share of federal transfers to urban municipalities throughout the state. Mayor Juraci Magalhães was thus in a position to use city funds to support the health care program once he gave it his approval. Magalhães was a prominent doctor in Fortaleza who had been in private practice for much of his life and had run a small pharmaceutical laboratory in the city. His training as a doctor and experience in the medical field meant that his approval of the Farmácia Viva program was doubly significant, for he was able not only to support the program financially as the mayor but also to legitimate the use of traditional medicine through the respect he had gained as a practicing doctor.

The significance of Magalhães's approval in decisions regarding health services cannot be underestimated in relation to the creation of Farmácia Viva. Almost all of the public health workers with whom I spoke acknowledged the support of Fortaleza's mayor for the program and were anxious that the upcoming elections might jeopardize its future should a new mayor be elected. The connection between politics and health was never more explicitly expressed than when public health workers assured me that the only reason the program had found favor was that Magalhães was such a strong proponent of it and that a new administration might decide to abandon this program in favor of something else.

Aside from strengthening the position of the mayor with respect to health care allocations, it is also important to note that the process of municipalization of health care funding strengthened the relationship of the university system to the public health care sector. Immediately following the decision to municipalize funding, the Universidade Federal do Ceará agreed to put its academic infrastructure and human resources at the disposal of the city of Fortaleza and surrounding municipalities. The university responded to specific requests made by the municipalities in the areas of health education and research and became a partner in defining problems and potential solutions for the municipalities as well as offering to train various health care personnel (Kisil and Tancredi 1996, 398).[4] It was precisely through this connection between the Universidade Federal and the public health system that the Farmácia Viva program was able to secure the help of scientists to analyze medicinal plants and to produce some of the traditional remedies sold at the program's clinics. The link between research science and medicinal plants also profoundly shaped the way Farmácia Viva presented traditional medicine.

In sum, the shift toward municipalization instigated by the Sistema Único de Saúde allowed the city of Fortaleza to respond to the health care needs of its low-income communities with greater financial and technical flexibility. The increased power of the mayor over health care matters and the involvement of the university's resources and expertise in turn forged new relationships between local officials, university scientists, and public health workers who were instrumental in developing the Farmácia Viva program and in reshaping the cultural categories associated with traditional medicine.

Although the emergence of Farmácia Viva can be traced back to the national health care reforms and to the local structural changes made in response to the reforms, the guiding principles of the program itself were largely influenced by the ideology of international medical development work. In particular, the concept of using traditional medicine to meet basic health care needs of low-income communities was adopted directly from the global health policy directives outlined by the World Health Organization in the late 1970s.

In 1978 the World Health Organization (WHO) adopted the goal of "health for all by the year 2000" and cited the need for worldwide access to a comprehensive primary health care system (Bryant 1980, 382). According to this new mandate, medical development was to be organized, directed, and regulated by a systemization of health care resources in developing countries, with the WHO as the ultimate overseer of the program. In a 1980 article describing the movement, John Bryant, a deputy assistant secretary for international health for the U.S. Department of Health, Education, and Welfare, summarized the fundamental ideas of the health for all concept as including

- Appropriate technology, that is the recognition of the limitations and disadvantages of high technology and the importance of less complex, lower cost technology appropriate to local needs and capabilities
- Awareness of the distorting effects of an over-emphasis on curative medicine, especially on hospital-based, specialty-oriented, technologically sophisticated care, and consequent emphasis on more balanced approaches to prevention and to lower cost, technologically simplified modes of medical care
- The emergence of primary health care, emphasizing preventive, promotive and curative services available at or very close to communities in culturally acceptable patterns, and at locally affordable costs
- Encouragement of developing nations to scientifically research and utilize medicinal plants (383)

The influence of international health directives on health care projects in developing countries has been widely noted by medical anthropologists and critical scholars of development (Escobar 1995, Ferguson 1990, Morgan 1993, Scheper-Hughes 1992). In the case of Farmácia Viva, public health workers repeated many of the more general directives of the WHO verbatim, explaining that less complex, low-cost technology was often more appropriate to the needs of people in communities such as Pirambu. One of the directors of the program, Eugina Francesca da Luz, told me, "The Farmácia Viva program was so important because it replicated people's culturally accepted notions of health care." In response to my queries about the use of medicinal plants, she assured me, "Don't worry, we have the approval of the WHO. They strongly support the use of traditional medicine." Even the educational material for the program displayed the WHO's then nearly out-of-date slogan "health for all by the year 2000."

By far the most important of the WHO's directives in terms of Farmácia Viva was the dictate to "encourage developing nations to scientifically research and utilize medicinal plants." The directive can be read as a kind of technical solution addressed to the preceding four WHO statements. If as the WHO suggested, "appropriately low technology" should be valued over "high-tech, curative approaches to medicine" and if this technology should further be presented in "culturally acceptable patterns," then traditional medicinal systems become a useful aid in achieving the goal of health for all by 2000. However, I want to look more closely at this and other WHO mandates, as it was not just any kind of traditional medicine that developing countries were encouraged to use; rather, they were being encouraged to promote a highly specific kind of medicinal plant use.

In a 1987 article titled "The Best of Both Worlds: Bringing Traditional Medicine Up to Date," WHO staff member Olayiwola Akerele noted that "the WHO is mandated to ensure that what is of value in local communities' traditional systems of medicine is made use of in the health services" (177). The key question is what was considered to be of value by the WHO. Akerele goes on to remind his readers that "past experience shows that many valuable drugs have been derived from plants and information that is utilized in traditional medicine is often an indication that is worth scientific study" (179). According to Akerele, then, what had value to the WHO were medicinal plants that could be proven effective by science and that could possibly lead to the production of profitable pharmaceutical drugs.[5]

To capture the potential value of medicinal plants, Akerele advises that "traditional medicine be put on a scientific basis" by

- Critical examination of traditional material medicine and practices
- Accurate identification of plants and other natural products used
- Identification of useful remedies and practices and suppression of those that are partly ineffective or unsafe (178)

He then asserts,

Nationals with responsibilities for drug quality control and with advanced degrees in chemistry or pharmacy have been trained to select the best methods of assaying and standardizing medicinal plant extracts and to prepare standard protocols of chemical or bioassay methods. The aim is to improve the efficacy and safety of remedies derived from medicinal plants, many of which contain pharmacologically active agents that in an overdose may have harmful effects. (178)

Part of what Akerele is suggesting here is that a conceptual shift can be made from thinking about medicinal plants within a local, cultural framework to thinking about and acting upon them within an abstract, scientific framework in which the effects of medicinal plants can be compared to those of pharmaceutical drugs. Standardizing medicinal plants requires having an advanced degree in chemistry or pharmacy, and standard protocols of chemical or bioassay methods should be used. Likewise noteworthy, terms such as "pharmacologically active agents" and "overdose" normally reserved for pharmaceuticals are used to describe the actions of medicinal plants. According to the WHO, then, the kind of traditional medicine that should be promoted in developing countries is the kind that can most readily be made to resemble pharmaceuticals.

I want to be clear that my point here is not that the WHO mandates regarding the scientific study of traditional knowledge represent a new commitment on the part of scientists to investigate the scientific properties of medicinal plants. Naturalists, botanists, physicians, and other scholars have studied the medicinal properties of plants for hundreds of years. In 1875 Agostinho Vieira de Mattos, a physician in Rio de Janeiro, studied the *quina-da-serra* used popularly in Brazil as an antimalarial and general antithermic. He isolated from its bark a bitter material that he called *vieirine*. Several years later, Domingos José Freire, a professor of organic chemistry at a medical school in Rio de Janeiro, undertook the chemical study of *vieirine* and found it was of acidic nature and not an alkaloid (Mors 1997, 310). These nineteenth-century studies and hundreds of others like them show clearly that the abstraction of plants into a scientific framework and the attempt to detail their physiological affects on the body are not twentieth-century innovations. What is novel about the WHO's mandates is thus not that they place medicinal plants within a scientific framework but rather that they suggest that medicinal plants can be compared to and treated like a genuinely twentieth-century innovation—synthetic drugs.

Synthetic pharmaceuticals were developed soon after World War II, and their arrival drastically curtailed the use of plant-derived medicines. It not only curtailed the use of plant-derived medicines but also— and perhaps more importantly—the use of a whole host of products for which medicinal properties were claimed. During the 1800s and on through the early 1900s the sales of tonics, elixirs, and nostrums were rampant in Brazil and the United States. Because there were so few controls on medicine and because the general public did not yet have a firmly established category for what a drug should be, such products found many enthusiastic consumers. However, once synthetic drugs were introduced and the "drug" category became more firmly defined as something that had to be manufactured according to governmental regulations, came in distinct packaging, and required a doctor's prescription, it became much more difficult to sell pseudomedicines. The legitimation of the drug category can then in some important ways be seen to depend upon the exclusion of everything that is not a drug. Arguably the main point of this exclusionary process was to target and eliminate the pseudomedicines, but in so doing, medicinal plants, ironically the very foundation of synthetic drugs, were excluded as well. Only once the authority of synthetic drugs was well established and the category of "drug" well defined could organizations like the WHO begin to call for the use of medicinal plants, as there was now no threat that they would destabilize the drug category. The fascinating aspect of the WHO's promotion of traditional medicine is that it is now being used to familiarize people with the categories associated with synthetic drugs.

Significantly, the development of pharmaceuticals consolidated the cultural category of "drug" as an object that was manufactured; that had an active ingredient, a purity level, and a Latin name; that came in distinct packaging such as bottles, pills, capsules, and tubes, accompanied by a list of required dosages, warnings, and contraindications; that had to be prescribed by an authority; and that had to be sold at specific sites.

This was a "drug" in its ideal typical form, and it was this framework and all the cultural practices it entailed that could now be reapplied to medicinal plants.

With the expansion of the pharmaceutical industry, pharmaceutical companies began the search for medicinal plants that could become the basis for new, highly profitable drugs. One of the first groups to take up this search was the U.S. National Cancer Institute (NCI), a part of the National Institutes of Health. In 1960 the NCI initiated a program to search for plants that could lead to anticancer drugs (Aseby 1997). A small number of pharmaceutical companies had established natural-product screening divisions in the 1950s, with more following suit after the NIH established its program. The increased willingness of pharmaceutical companies to evaluate medicinal plants within the framework of synthetic drugs encouraged the international development community to consider traditional medicine as a possible solution for providing low-cost, preventive medical care to low-income communities in developing countries.

Thus when, in the late 1970s, the WHO began to call for an integration between traditional medicine and biomedicine, and started to lobby for the use of traditional medicinal systems, it did so not with the intention of promoting a return to the extant systems of traditional knowledge but rather with the explicit recognition that the kind of traditional medicine it was going to promote was actually biomedicine.[6]

Although this biomedicalized approach to traditional medicine formed the core of the Farmácia Viva program, the health care workers associated with the program consistently described their work as being an alternative to biomedicine rather than a less capital-intensive version of it. The technical program coordinator, Dr. Eufrazina Lopes, stressed, "Farmácia Viva offers an alternative to the fancy clinical medical regimes of the rich. Learning to use our medicinal plants is better because it's something poor residents can then grow at home, and they won't have to rely as much on pharmaceuticals." In a similar vein, Reinaldo César, an agronomist at the *horto municipal*, the program's central garden for medicinal plants, told me, "I do this work from my heart because it is a great cycle, growing the plants and then offering a natural remedy for the poor to use in place of pharmaceuticals. It gives me great pride."

Health care workers consistently called attention to Farmácia Viva's use of "culturally authentic" medicine and emphasized that it validated low-income residents' extant forms of knowledge. And they often counterposed their own knowledge of biomedicine to that of residents who possessed knowledge about traditional medicine. A public health worker for the program said, "We understand the western system of biomedicine, but they [residents] have medical knowledge that is important to validate as well." When I asked him to clarify this point, he said, "We can show respect for their culture by demonstrating that some of their medical knowledge is true."

Another factor in favor of Farmácia Viva noted by a health care worker was favela residents' fear of hospitals: "The people we see often find hospitals in Fortaleza alienating. It's not what they're used to, but coming to a clinic where they actually have traditional medicine—recipes that they are familiar with or that they saw their grandparents use—this sets them at ease."

Health care workers' interpretations of their own program offer insights into the images that middle- and upper-middle-class city residents hold of Fortaleza's lower classes. Understood as residents making a difficult transition from the rural interior and still being attached to their prior lives in a myriad of complicated ways, health care workers for Farmácia Viva deemed it appropriate to supply favela residents with the familiar feeling of traditional medicine.

As was pointed out to me by the doctor leading the health council meetings, however, the people of Pirambu were often more interested in explicit forms of western biomedicine than they were in preventive medical practices, let alone traditional ones. In fact, as scholars have found, biomedical services have become yet another indicator of class status in Brazil (Béhague, Gonçalves, and Dias da Costa 2002; Edmonds 2007, 2010; Sanabria 2010). Older residents of the favela often had moved to Fortaleza specifically to gain increased access to a broad range of urban amenities, including what they perceived as technologically advanced health care, while younger residents were beginning to aspire to privatized forms of biomedical care.

The misrecognition of favela residents as desiring tradition and thus as somehow needing or being more comfortable with traditional medicine glosses over another possible reading of the promotion of traditional medicine that I have been describing: in Fortaleza, government management of traditional medicine takes the particular form of redeploying it as a kind of pharmaceutical drug. In the process of exercising this form of management, the Farmácia Viva program offers a fascinating opportunity to observe how the cultural categories associated with pharmaceutical drugs are reinstantiated in the context of traditional medicine and thereby simultaneously are transforming it. In this sense, the terms "traditional knowledge" and "medicinal plants" have a new referent; they point to the creation of a hybrid object, a plant/drug, whose origins were grounded in national health care reform that changed local health care politics and in international development directives that brought about a shift in the status of traditional medicine.

Local Plants for Local Peoples

By the time I arrived in the field in September 1998, the Farmácia Viva program had been running strong for more than six years. From the beginning it received backing from two mayors representing different political parties and was expected to continue receiving financial and technical support from the municipal government for the foreseeable future. Since its inception, the program's slogan has been "Local Plants for Local Peoples," which captures the program's essential message that local plants and medicinal remedies can effectively be used to treat the basic health needs of low-income, local people.

What this slogan effectively erases, however, is the work that is needed to transform local plants into effective medicine. As I argue above, to count as effective medicine, traditional medicine must first be abstracted into a scientific paradigm, evaluated according to certain criteria promoted by the WHO, and then be made to look as much as possible like pharmaceutical drugs. City government and health officials in Fortaleza accomplished these tasks by adhering to particular social practices such as choosing specific kinds of plants, adopting a formal registration process for medicinal plants designed to mimic pharmaceutical registration, and creating traditional medicinal products that mimicked the forms associated with pharmaceuticals.

The first phase of transforming traditional medicine involved the selection of the plants themselves. The plants used in the program, some twenty-five of them, were chosen by scientists at the Laboratório de Fitoterápicos e Homeopáticos (Natural Products Laboratory at the Universidade Federal do Ceará). While many of the plants like *acerola* and *mentrasto* are native to Ceará, others including *poejo* have been specifically introduced for use in the program.

Soon after my arrival in the field I met with program cofounder Francisco Abreu Matos to learn more about the plants used by Farmácia Viva. Dr. Abreu Matos was the director of the Natural Products Laboratory. He had lived in Fortaleza all of his life and was a pharmacologist by training. At this stage in my fieldwork, I was still trying to determine how the program identified which medicinal plants to use. I pressed Dr. Abreu Matos about where his scientists collected information on the local medicinal plants. "Did you conduct interviews? Consult local shamans? Pay people for their great-aunt's medicinal collection?" I asked.

Dr. Abreu Matos gently shook his head and replied, "No, no, dear. You don't seem to understand, these people. Why, they don't even know half the time what they are using. No, people are not the best source at all. The most reliable information about medicinal plants comes from ethnobotanical literature and from botanists who have recorded their findings." He continued, perhaps unsure if I was satisfied, "The knowledge about medicinal plants is really what we would call general knowledge. It belongs to nobody."

There is a certain political benefit to flagging traditional knowledge as general knowledge, for by doing so it is conceptualized as being part of the national public domain rather than as belonging to a specific individual or community. Anthropologist Cori Hayden, writing about the International Cooperative Biodiversity Groups (ICBG) program, notes that scientists in Mexico have explicitly sought out medicinal plants in the public domain—found at markets and on highway shoulders and described in ethnobotanical literature—because they represent a kind of traditional knowledge that offers the easiest path to compliance with the 1992 United Nations Convention on Biological Diversity (CBD), which states that indigenous or local communities are entitled to just compensation for the use of their biological and intellectual resources. Though the politics of labeling the traditional knowledge and medicinal plants used in the Farmácia Viva program as "general knowledge" are of a different order than those of the Mexican scientists attempting to facilitate compliance with the CBD, in both cases categorizing medicinal plants as part of the general knowledge base serves the purpose of disconnecting plants and knowledge from social communities.

Plants that are already displaced from their social context are in turn more easily transformed into their new role as effective medicinal plants, for plants that are associated with the social knowledge of particular communities bear the stamp of that knowledge. A resident of Pirambu visiting a Farmácia Viva clinic might say, "My grandmother always used *mentrasto* with *agrião bravo* to cure tooth infections." Part of the point of both the WHO directives and the Farmácia Viva program is precisely to strip the plants clean of this kind of local knowledge, which may or may not be scientifically valid, and to replace it with scientific knowledge—the plant's toxicity level, purity ratios, and active ingredient—whose authority cannot be questioned. Thus representing plants as not having specific links to communities and viewing them as already free from those social relations makes the reshaping of medicinal plants as effective medicine that much easier.

The second phase of transforming traditional medicine into an effective form of medicine took place in Fortaleza at the Centro para o Desenvolvimento e Produção de Fitoterápicos (Center for the Technological Development and Production of Natural Medicine), where the medicinal plants used in the program were officially registered by city and public health officials. The center was located in a small office on the seventh floor of the Secretaria Municipal de Desenvolvimento Social (City Department of Social Development) that since the restructuring of the city's health care system housed the local offices of the state health department and its educational components. The office was situated, not coincidentally, just down the hall from an office bearing the name Centro de Registro e Desenvolvimento de Produtos Farmacêuticos (Center for the Registration and Development of Pharmaceutical Products). The location of Farmácia Viva's main office represents another connection between pharmaceuticals and medicinal plants, identifying *fitoterapia* as another form of biomedicine.

During one of my first visits to the Farmácia Viva office, its coordinator, Dr. Lopes, stated that one of the office's more important responsibilities was the official registration of the medicinal plants used in the program. To accomplish this, the staff followed the guidelines outlined in a booklet titled *Registro de medicamentos fitoterápicos* (Registry of natural medicines). The booklet, which the City of Fortaleza published in 1998, begins with an acknowledgment of World Health Organization standards: "The WHO recommends the use of plants as a therapeutic option, providing that their use has been selected according to scientific principles and is proven to be an effective therapeutic option" (3).

The pamphlet draws a distinction between "medicamento fitoterápico tradicional" (traditional medicinal plant use) and "medicamento fitoterápico novo" (new medicinal plant). Traditional medicinal plant use is defined as "medicinal plants used in the popular tradition without the evidence, knowledge, or information, of the health risks involved in its use" (4). New medicinal plant use is defined as "using plants whose safety and quality has been proven by scientific experiment, and whose active ingredient is known, and that have been registered for formal use by the city of Fortaleza" (5).

Here, a new form of traditional knowledge is being introduced that is implicitly linked to the city's official system of biomedicine. Unlike the old form of traditional medicine, the pamphlet promises that new traditional medicine will be safe and effective. The pamphlet also implies that in order for traditional medicine to be effective, it must have an active ingredient like pharmaceutical drugs do and that its use must be authorized by the city of Fortaleza.

To transform traditional medicinal plant use into the new and effective form of traditional medicine, health officials are expected to follow certain steps.[7] First the pamphlet advises, "One must identify the plant's official botanical name. Its genre, species, and variety should also be identified." Once the plant has been properly identified, its traditional nomenclature should be noted but not used. Next, the pamphlet states, "One must identify the part of the plant that has medicinal value and perform tests of authenticity in order to identify its active pharmacological ingredient. After the essence of the plant has been identified, then tests of purity and integrity should be performed on it in accordance with the criteria recommended by the World Health Organization" (7). The pamphlet states that documentation about the plant must be presented to the federal Ministry of the Environment, the Ministry of Agriculture, and the Empresa Brasileira de Pesquisa Agropecuaria (Embrapa), Brazil's largest state-run biotechnology company.[8]

The process of transforming traditional medicinal plant use into effective medicinal plant use is depicted as depending upon abstracting the plants into a scientific framework, by identifying their scientific name, performing tests to determine their toxicity levels, and identifying their active ingredients. These acts, all of which are aligned with the canonical category of "drug," also work to exclude the kinds of traditional medicine that cannot measure up to the standards associated with pharmaceutical drugs. If an active ingredient cannot be found in a particular plant, then regardless of its reputation among local users, it cannot be included in the repertoire of medicinal plants promoted by Farmácia Viva. In this way, only a very narrow subsection of traditional medicine is being authorized for use, based exclusively on its ability to be abstracted into a scientific framework and to mimic pharmaceutical properties.

In a pamphlet produced by the Center for the Technological Development and Production of Natural Medicine, the *Guia Fitoterápicos* (Natural medicine guide), the now legitimated effective medicinal plants are further linked to pharmaceutical drugs by describing them and the products made from them in terms that closely resemble those associated with biomedicine. The twenty-four medicinal plants discussed in the pamphlet are first grouped by "therapeutic specialty." Medicinal plants such as *capim santo* (a local grass) and *maracujá* (passion fruit) are placed in the category of plants with ingredients that act on the central nervous system, while *colônia* is listed as being one of the only plants effective for treating the cardiovascular system.

The grouping of plants by the actions they perform on bodily systems is particularly interesting because doing so reinforces biomedical rather than local understandings of how medicinal plants work. In Pirambu, when I asked about the use of a specific medicinal plant, I was told it was "good for colds and flus" or that it "helped reduce nervousness." In the pamphlet, the plants are described as acting not on general ailments or even on specific parts of the body but rather on large bodily systems such as the central nervous system or the digestive system. While the idea of the body as an entity composed of biological systems that reacts chemically to the substances it imbibes is present in Pirambu, it is not typically associated with the way medicinal plants interact with the body. By ascribing these kinds of biomedically based actions to medicinal plants, the pamphlet frames them as a kind of pharmaceutical drug and simultaneously naturalizes biomedical descriptions of the body.

In the next section of the pamphlet, descriptions are provided of each of the ten medicinal products that are made by Farmácia Viva's laboratories. By examining the pictures of these products and their descriptions, one can see that the products' distinctive packaging and warning labels have been designed to closely mimic those associated with pharmaceutical drugs.

One of the first products depicted is *capsulas de hortelã rasteira*. The capsules, filled with ground leaves of *hortelã rasteira*, a mint, are used to treat gastrointestinal disorders such as diarrhea. The product comes in a small, plastic bottle with a childproof cap, such as you would find in a standard drugstore. A label, which has been pasted on slightly askew, notes the name of the product and indicates fabrication and validation dates. At the top of the label is the statement "Made by Farmácia Viva, in accordance with the Health Department of Fortaleza."

Unlike in Pirambu, where I often witnessed the use of *hortelã* tea to soothe the stomach, the Farmácia Viva version of the medicine consisted of leaves ground into a powder and placed in capsules. The use of capsules is significant because capsules are one of the most salient features of a drug and differentiate pharmaceutical drugs from local remedies used in Pirambu. By presenting *hortelã rasteira* in capsule form, Farmácia Viva effectively recasts traditional medicine as a kind of pharmaceutical medicine.

The validation date on the product's bottle as well as the stamp of approval from the city health department are two more features common to pharmaceutical drugs that have now been linked to effective forms of traditional medicine. The health department's approval is particularly striking because it suggests that in order for traditional medicine to be legitimate it must secure the approval of health care authorities within the biomedical establishment.

In addition to a picture of the product itself, the pamphlet includes the text of the warning label that comes with all of Farmácia Viva's medicinal products. The label describes the *hortelã rasteira* medicine in the following manner: "30 gelatin capsules, containing 200 mg of dry leaves of Mentha x villosa." Following this description, "indicações" (indications) are presented describing the various symptoms that would lead one to try this drug. Then, "precauções e contra-indicações" (precautions and contraindications) are listed, including the advice that one should not take the medicine while one is pregnant. Next, "interações medicamentos" (drug interactions) are listed, stressing that medicinal plants, like other drugs, do interact with other medications. Finally, possible adverse reactions to the plants are listed and patients are directed to contact a doctor if they begin to feel ill after taking the medications.

All of these warnings suggest that traditional medicine can and in fact should be thought about within the framework of pharmaceutical drugs. Thus, the same warnings that apply to pharmaceutical drugs should also be applied to medicinal plants and the remedies that are made from them. Attaching warnings to the Farmácia Viva products also implies that in order for traditional medicine to be safe and effective, certain guidelines, akin to those applied to pharmaceuticals, must be followed.

The social practices I have described enable the Farmácia Viva program to transform traditional medicinal use into effective medicinal plant use, a category that closely resembles that of pharmaceutical medication. By carefully selecting the medicinal plants, abstracting them into a scientific framework, formally registering them, and manufacturing them with distinct packaging and warning labels that resemble pharmaceutical drugs, a new object was created, one that could now be understood by government officials, university scientists, medical doctors, and even biotechnology firms. This new object, "the effective medicinal plant"—what I might refer to as a hybrid plant/drug—can then be used by health care officials as a vehicle through which to educate residents of communities like Pirambu that there is really only one standard against which all forms of medicine, including the local medicinal practices with which they are familiar, could be measured—that of biomedicine.

Caution: Medicinal Plants Are Drugs!

Having transformed a select group of traditional medicinal plants into effective forms of medicine according to the guidelines prescribed by the Farmácia Viva program, the second and more monumental task that Fortaleza health officials faced was to convince residents of low-income communities that the local medical practices they were accustomed to following should be replaced by a similar but more effective form of traditional medicine. Health officials attempted to accomplish this formidable challenge by contesting local residents' authority over traditional medicine, arguing that, if understood properly, it closely resembled biomedicine, and thus its practice required the intervention of medical authorities.

Soon after my arrival in Fortaleza in 1998, I visited several of the local health clinics scattered throughout Pirambu and noticed a series of brightly colored posters listing the dangers of medicinal plants. The posters were put out by the City Department of Social Development, the Coordenadoria da Saúde (a health services coordinating office), and the Pharmaceutical Aid Center. At the top of all the posters was the same warning in large, yellow letters—"CAUTION!"—followed by the question "Are you using your medicinal plants correctly?" Below the question, each poster had an illustration of a generic medicinal plant, and attached to each leaf was a warning about the dangers of medicinal plants: "ATTENTION: Just because they are natural doesn't mean they're safe! The incorrect use of medicinal plants can be dangerous!" And "It is important to know the correct manner of preparing plants." And "If you are pregnant, don't use medicinal plants without a doctor's direction." And finally, "If you don't get better with medicinal plants seek a doctor!"

The warnings attempt to draw a distinction between the correct and incorrect usage of medicinal plants and implicitly assert that the authors of the poster—and the health officials, scientists, and medical doctors with whom they are allied—have the authority to prescribe the correct traditional medicine practices rather than the residents of Pirambu. The phrase "It is important to know the correct manner of preparing plants" does the double work of warning residents that there is a particular method by which these plants should be prepared and that it is the health authorities who know what that correct manner is.

The caution that medicinal plants cannot be considered safe just because they are natural is another attempt to weaken residents' authority over traditional medicine. Here, the term "natural" can be understood as signifying not just organic but also familiar, culturally acceptable, and authentic, for residents of Pirambu do view traditional medicine as natural in the sense that it is a time-worn, at-hand, and immanently local practice. What the posters imply, then, is that just because residents are accustomed to following traditional medical practices doesn't mean doing so is safe and that to avoid risk they will need to modify their use of traditional medicine according to the methods prescribed by public health authorities.

The final warning, to seek help from a doctor if the plant medicine doesn't work, is the posters' most explicit wording to shift authority over traditional medicine away from residents and put it into the hands of health authorities. The message the posters deliver is that even if residents treat themselves with traditional medicine, clinical doctors have the ultimate authority over how that medicine will interact with the human body.

Brochures that were handed out by public health workers likewise were quite explicit about the necessity of avoiding risks when practicing traditional medicine. All of the brochures that were handed out at the health units and during public health workers' home visits had a list of places where one could find "safe" medicinal plants in Fortaleza. The list included the municipal garden, the state Department of Agriculture, the health department, the health center in the Jardim das Oliveiras neighborhood, and several state hospitals.

Yet access to medicinal plants is not confined to the short list of locations sanctioned by the city of Fortaleza. Residents of the city's favelas can purchase them at nearly all of the local grocery stores that dot the favela, at the open-air markets in town, and from roadside vendors who sell a wide array of herbs and other plants. What the brochures make clear, however, is that there are only certain locations from which it is safe to purchase medicinal plants and that there is a health risk attached to purchasing medicinal plants at any other location. By creating official social spaces for the sale of medicinal plants, the municipal government further identifies the plants with drugs, for just as with pharmaceutical drugs, the safe consumption of herbal remedies depends upon purchasing them from a location formally designated for that purpose.

People not only purchase medicinal plants, however; they also grow them. Nearly all of the houses I visited in Pirambu had at least a small batch of medicinal plants growing in their windowsills, buckets, or recycled plastic bottles. Here again, the government brochures define this behavior as risky. The brochures start by asserting that people need to know the origin of the medicinal plants and not to grow plants in polluted locations. In particular, they warn that to safely grow medicinal plants, residents must avoid polluted water and soil that is near a dump or a sewer or where animals roam.

What is remarkable about these seemingly simple, common-sense warnings is how difficult they would be for most residents to heed. Directions such as finding "water that isn't polluted" and "soil that doesn't have trash strewn around it" are nearly impossible for residents of the favela to follow. As residents themselves pointed out during the health council meetings, their homes often sit amid polluted water, sewers, dumps, and strewn trash. It can be a struggle to find not just clean spaces in which to safely grow medicinal plants but clean spaces in which to safely live at all. Like the doctor leading the health council meetings, though, government officials wanted not so much to remind residents of the daily risks of living on the margins of a rapidly growing urban city as to help diminish the gap between favela life and urban city life, something that in this case was partly accomplished by extending the standards and social practices associated with biomedicine to residents' practice of traditional medicine.

Other educational material handed out in the health units and by public health workers attempted to drive home similar messages in the form of comic strips. One of these, titled "Farmácia Viva," began by introducing readers to a benevolent scientist, Dr. Abreu Matos, who in turn introduced readers to two cartoon medicinal plants. He proceeded to take a walk with the plants through a medicinal plant garden and tell them about themselves and how they could be used appropriately. Throughout the story, links were made between medicinal plants and drugs. The comic book starts out with Dr. Abreu Matos introducing the two medicinal plants and explaining that they are called "medicinal" because they produce the same type of pharmacological action as drugs do. "Medicines made from parts of us," the little plants exclaim, "are known as *fitoterápicos*, or *plantas medicinais* [medicinal plants]."

Next, Dr. Abreu Matos invites the plants outside to see a living pharmacy, a garden where their many friends and relatives are growing. Here again it is emphasized that a garden must be created in a clean place, away from dumps, sewers, pigsties, and the edges of roads. Dr. Abreu Matos also advises that ideally every household should have a medicinal plant garden because medicinal plants are easy to prepare and cheaper and less risky than pharmaceuticals if used correctly.

Once the comic strip has introduced readers to the concept of medicinal plants and instructed them on how to grow the plants, it then advises readers that there are certain risks associated with them. Here, the cartoon plants break out into sounds of alarm: "CAUTIONS???" they cry, looking horrified. "Why do we need those?" "Because," Dr. Abreu Matos explains, "just because you are natural doesn't mean you are safe. The incorrect use of medicinal plants is DANGEROUS." The plants exclaim, "DANGEROUS! How could we be dangerous?" "Don't worry," says Dr. Abreu Matos soothingly, "medicinal plants are only DRUGS, when used correctly and with adequate instruction." He then lists some of the precautions mentioned in the posters, including that medicinal plants should be grown or purchased only in particular locations and not collected from dirty streams or polluted places, that people should know which medicinal plants are toxic, should not mix medicinal plant remedies with one another, and consult a doctor if they don't get better. He also warns that if people make the remedies themselves, they must use them within five days and write down the name of the plant and the date it was used.

Here again, the comic book clearly promotes the use of medicinal plants according to standards generally associated with pharmaceutical drugs. Directions such as using the herbal remedies within a five-day period tend to normalize the concept that medicinal plants, like pharmaceuticals, have expiration dates and that the safe use of homemade remedies depends upon adhering to those dates. Similarly, the warning to consult a doctor if the herbal remedy doesn't work insinuates that a clinical doctor has the ultimate authority over knowledge about traditional medicine rather than a friend or family member.

Following the list of instructions to carefully use medicinal plants, the comic strip discusses what makes the plants effective. "Do you know," Dr. Abreu Matos asks the medicinal plants, "what an active ingredient is?" One of the plants responds correctly that it is "one or more substances that exist in plants and produce the desired effect to obtain a cure." "But why would this be important?" they ask. "Because," asserts Dr. Abreu Matos, "in order for people to use your leaves as medicine, you must be sure that you have an active ingredient that is safe. If you do, then you can impress your friends!" Dr. Abreu Matos lists fourteen plants that have been tested by his lab and found safe. The scientific name and the active ingredient of each plant is provided, as well as directions about how to use it correctly.

Suggesting that medicinal plants have active ingredients and that the active ingredient is in fact the very essence of each plant is perhaps the most explicit link that the educational material makes between medicinal plants and drugs. By attributing the efficacy of a medicinal plant to a single ingredient that can only be identified by a medical doctor, scientist, or public health authority, the comic book effectively delegitimizes local explanations of efficacy. Here again, the health officials' construction of medicinal plants as pharmaceutical drugs works to ensure that it is they who can dictate the correct use of traditional medicine rather than residents of communities like Pirambu.

Warnings about the risks of traditional medicine have even permeated standard public health comic books designed to teach lower-income populations about basic health problems. In one comic book a woman is in a local pharmacy trying to buy some pills for a stomach ache. The clerk attempts to take advantage of her by giving her the wrong medicine and overcharging her; however, she is soon rescued by a pharmacist who warns her about the proper way to purchase and use pharmaceuticals. He then asserts, "It is important to remember that these warnings go for medicinal plants as well." "Medicinal plants as well?" the woman asks, a look of dismay on her face. "But aren't they natural?" "Yes they are," responds the pharmacist, "but using them in the wrong form is dangerous!" "Remember," he exhorts, "medicinal plants must be used according to the correct procedures." The pamphlet concludes by providing a list of the warnings repeated in the other brochures and posters.

What all of these educational pamphlets and comic books have in common is that they promote the application of a set of formal standards to the use of traditional medicine by calling attention to the ways medicinal plants and remedies resemble pharmaceutical drugs. As I have argued, this resemblance was deliberately constructed through the work of scientists and city officials to transform medicinal plants into effective medicine. Once the effective form of traditional medicine had been distinguished from traditional medicine, public health officials could then argue that a new set of social practices should be applied to its use. By drawing attention to the similarities in the components of traditional medicinal remedies and standard pharmaceutical drugs, the Farmácia

Viva program has sought to co-opt traditional medicine as a realm of knowledge and practice over which the medical establishment has the ultimate authority.

Specifically, the intention was for residents to learn that what makes traditional medicine effective is that it resembles pharmaceutical drugs and that due to this resemblance it must be practiced according to the same set of guidelines—taken in specific dosages, not mixed with other medications, not used during pregnancy, and sometimes requiring the guidance of a doctor—that apply to biomedicine. In establishing new forms of authority over traditional medicine, the educational material was produced to normalize the forms, practices, and cultural categories of pharmaceutical drugs by inserting them into the practice of traditional medicine. Next I explore how a similar process was accomplished through patient-doctor interactions at Farmácia Viva's traditional medicine clinics.

Clinic Visits: Prescribing Knowledge

In accordance with Farmácia Viva's mandates, three medical clinics were established to educate residents of low-income communities about the correct usage of medicinal plants. Two of these clinics were combined with state-funded clinics already situated in low-income neighborhoods to provide general health care services. The third clinic was connected to the Federal University of Ceará and devoted entirely to instruction in traditional medicine. I observed these clinics on four or five occasions, and I want to present several examples of how doctors sought to transform patients' ideas about traditional medicine in order to illustrate how new conceptual categories and social practices were created in the process.

The first clinic I visited was the Clínica Água Fria. Situated just outside of the Federal University of Ceará campus, the clinic served a large favela with a population of about fifteen thousand that had grown up along the university's west side. Behind the modest block of buildings that comprised the clinic, a small medicinal garden had been planted to grow the plants that would be given away for free to visiting patients. The clinic was staffed by a group of volunteers from the university's social medicine program who were referred to as medical assistants and met with patients on a first come, first served basis. The client base for the clinic consisted primarily of the residents of the adjoining neighborhood in addition to any relatives and friends they might happen to bring with them.

One of the first patients to come to the clinic on the day I visited was a young woman named Rosa who brought with her a small baby girl. She sat down quietly, holding the child firmly to her chest. "My baby has the flu," Rosa told the clinic worker. "She's had it for a week now, and it's too long. She's sick—she coughs all the time and she can't sleep."

The young medical assistant, Roberto, responded that it did indeed sound like her child had the flu and said he would give her something to stop her baby from coughing and help her get better, something that she could make at home. But first she had to listen to his directions very carefully, as otherwise the remedy wouldn't work. Rosa cautiously nodded her head and looked curiously at the packets of plants and mimeographed instructions that Roberto was taking out of a drawer.

"Here," he said when he had the necessary products assembled. "This is what you do: you mix the *malvarico*, *mentrasto*, and *alecrim pimenta* in a pot—be careful to wash them first [because] these are from the garden. Then you boil them with water and drain that off—that's very important—then refill the pot with water and boil them again, this time with three cups of sugar. Keep it boiling until it forms a syrup and most of the water is gone. The syrup that's left is what you'll use to give to your baby."

Throughout this explanation Rosa nodded her head in agreement. Now she smiled at Roberto and pointed at the plants, exclaiming, "That's what my aunt always makes!"

Roberto grinned widely. "Exactly," he said. "That's exactly right."

"But," continued Rosa, "she doesn't make it like that."

"No?" asked Roberto, somewhat apprehensively.

"No, she doesn't make the plants boil twice, and she doesn't use this one," she said, pointing to the *alecrim pimenta*.

Roberto picked up the small clump of leaves and said, "*Alecrim pimenta* is very important. It's what's going to help your baby's cough. It's also important to boil the plants first, before you add the sugar. That's what makes them clean and safe to use as medicine."

Rosa nodded her head somewhat doubtfully, but swinging her baby onto her back she carefully picked up the plants and clutched the free medicine in her hands, thanking Roberto for his help.

"If you have a problem," Roberto added, "be sure to come back to the clinic immediately, and remember to follow all the steps we talked about. The directions are on the sheet of paper. If you can't remember something, look at the sheet. Your baby's going to get better."

Rosa smiled at this. "If God wills it," she said simply and made her way out the door.

After Rosa left Roberto remarked to me, "It's important to validate their own knowledge, to use the plants they do, but they have to learn to do it correctly. It has to be true."

In this instance what was true for Roberto and the institutions with which he was allied were medical treatments that could be proven to have scientific efficacy. The knowledge Rosa brought to the clinic visit about medicinal plants was only useful to Roberto to the extent that it provided a culturally acceptable vehicle for the delivery of scientific knowledge. Thus when Rosa pointed out that the remedy was familiar to her because she'd seen her aunt make something similar, she received positive validation from Roberto. However, when she began to challenge Roberto's authority by asserting that her aunt used a different combination of plants, he swiftly drew a distinction between the kind of local traditional medicine practiced by her aunt and the effective form of traditional medicine he was advocating in the clinic. In order for the medicine to be safe and effective, Rosa had to use the combination of plants prescribed by Roberto and to prepare the medicine according to his directions.

In prescribing a new set of directions for a medicinal plant already known as a home remedy, as happened with Rosa, a different category is created for effective traditional medicine, one that has its roots in state institutions, international health organizations, and ethnobotanical research. What is particularly important about this new category is that it derives its authority from a group of medical experts and a highly specific set of institutions rather than the local practitioners of traditional medicine.

A few weeks later I visited a second clinic, the Clínica Hugo da Frota Barroso Filho, on the edge of another low-income community in the southwest corner of the city. It was established by the state health department in 1986 to provide basic health care services to the surrounding population. In 1995 the clinic became part of the Farmácia Viva program, and a garden was located behind its facility as well as a small laboratory to produce medicinal products from the plants grown there. The five doctors practicing at the clinic were offered a short training course in *fitoterapia* and were asked to inform patients, when appropriate, about the option of using effective traditional medicine.

I arrived at the clinic in the middle of a hot afternoon, and much of the staff had already gone to lunch or taken an afternoon break. The only doctor on call was Luis Santos, a gynecologist, who kindly agreed to speak with me and later allowed me to observe him while he treated several patients.

Dr. Santos said he was originally from the interior of Ceará and moved to Fortaleza to study medicine. Before starting work at the Barroso Filho clinic in 1997, he worked at another government health clinic for nineteen years. He explained that at the Barroso Filho clinic the way the delivery of traditional medicine worked was that "if there is a natural equivalent for a pharmaceutical drug that could be taken in place of it, I offer that as an option for the patient. I first inform [them] that an option exists, that it doesn't have side effects, that it's totally natural, and that it's going to do exactly the same thing as the pharmaceutical drug will. Depending on what they say, I write a prescription for one of the medicinal products made here or for pharmaceuticals."

He informed me that only about 30 percent of the patients he sees choose a medication made from plants over standard pharmaceuticals. When I asked him why he thought the percentage was so low, he suggested that it was probably because there was not widespread advertising for medications based on medicinal plants as there was for pharmaceutical drugs.

Over the next few hours he allowed me to observe him as he treated patients. One of the first patients was Luisa, a woman in her late thirties who came to the clinic with complaints of severe menstrual cramps. He asked her some preliminary questions: Did she have any children? Yes, four. Was she working? Yes, she worked as a housecleaner two or three times a week in Fortaleza and occasionally took in wash for a couple of families in her neighborhood. Dr. Santos explained that there might be many reasons for her menstrual cramps including high blood pressure, stress, or a change in eating habits, or they might be an indication of something more serious—possibly she would need a hysterectomy. He wanted to make another appointment with Luisa so he could perform a full examination, and he asked her if she'd be willing to come back the following day. Luisa agreed, and they made an appointment for three o'clock.

Just as she was about to leave, Luisa mentioned offhand that she had also been experiencing vaginal itching and hadn't been able to find relief by using "the normal methods." Dr. Santos asked her what she was using as a treatment. "Well" replied Luisa, "I sometimes make a poultice of *confrei* [comfrey, a popular medicinal plant in Ceará and elsewhere] and *aroeira*, and I apply it at night. Or, if I can't find the *aroeira*, I'll just use the *confrei*."

Dr. Santos responded that there were several other things she could do that might be more effective. In the first place there was a pharmaceutical drug she could use, but there was also a natural cream that would be effective as well, *creme de aroeira*. "You might have heard of it," he added.

Luisa said she hadn't heard of it, but if he thought it would work, she would try it. Dr. Santos pulled a package with a skinny tube and a sheet of instructions down from a nearby shelf. Holding the package, he explained to Luisa, "You need to take it just like you would the creams you would buy at the drugstore. It's just as potent, and you should follow the directions carefully. You should apply it three times a day, placing just enough in the plastic tube to fill it. After you insert it, you need to carefully wash the tube in hot water and then place it back in the box."

Luisa looked slightly skeptically at the box and asked Dr. Santos if he was sure the medication would work. "Look," he told her soothingly, "there's a picture of the *aroeira* plant you used in your poultice right here on the label—you remember that, right? It's the same thing, only packaged in a tube instead. It'll be easier for you to use."

Luisa nodded at this and reached for the package. "And remember," Dr. Santos said as he handed it to her, "don't use the poultice any more when you're using this cream. It's not a good idea to mix medications." Again Luisa nodded and then asked the doctor if they were confirmed for the next day's appointment. He agreed, and they said goodbye.

After Luisa left, Dr. Santos commented that many women came to the clinic already having used medicinal plants or recognizing certain elements of the plant-based remedies the clinic provided, but what was important was that they learn the correct way to use medicinal plants. "Many doctors," he added, "aren't as willing as I am to incorporate popular medicine into their practice. They think the old customs should just be forgotten about and only pharmaceuticals should be prescribed. I don't have a problem with it, though. I don't think it can hurt."

I asked Dr. Santos if traditional medicine had comprised a part of his training as a medical student, and he responded that when he was a student, nearly twenty years earlier, no courses were offered in the treatment of patients with medicinal plants, but nowadays, because traditional medicine had become more valued, it was being incorporated into medical students' training at the Federal University.

Before leaving I asked him if he envisioned these popular remedies being used in the long term or if they would eventually be replaced by pharmaceuticals.

"I don't think it's a solution for the long term," he replied. "I myself almost never prescribe anything other than the *creme de aroeira* because this is the only thing I know of that really seems to work. Traditional medicine isn't practical or rapid enough to use in general. But it's nice to be able to offer a natural remedy occasionally."

"And what makes it natural?" I asked.

"Well," Dr. Santos replied, "because it's their medicine, really. I mean it's a popular remedy, and it's made from plants, besides."

His response, which linked "natural" with "popular remedies," again overlooked the steps that went into transforming the kinds of popular medicine found in the local communities surrounding Fortaleza into the versions of popular medicine offered at Farmácia Viva's clinics. Although clearly a distinction was drawn between local traditional medicine and clinic-sanctioned practices through the instructions that Dr. Santos gave about how to use one versus the other, once these forms were set against pharmaceutical drugs, the difference is erased and the medicinal practices constructed by Farmácia Viva become traditional medicine.

What I have been arguing here is that the form of medicine offered by Dr. Santos is in fact more firmly rooted in the social practices associated with pharmaceutical drugs than with those associated with traditional medicine. We can see this quite clearly in the interaction between Luisa and Dr. Santos. Luisa was in a doctor's office, being prescribed a medication. The medication itself, though made from plants, came in the kind of packaging generally associated with pharmaceuticals, a long, skinny tube accompanied by a plastic applicator and precise instructions. Luisa was instructed that the new form of traditional medication she received at the clinic shouldn't be mixed with other traditional medicinal remedies she may have used. By incorporating these social practices, all of which are commonly associated with biomedicine, into the practice of traditional medicine, the biomedical form and all that it entails—capital-intensive medical technology, a reliance on trained medical experts, biochemical understanding of the body—is itself extended.

Traditional Pharmaceuticals

I have argued that as part of local health care programming, itself made possible by new streams of funding from the SUS, the municipal government of Fortaleza has regulated and reorganized the production and consumption of traditional medicine on behalf of the city's low-income residents. Distinct from some health care professionals who characterized favela dwellers as marked by urban violence, the health care workers associated with Farmácia Viva conceptualized low-income residents as recent migrants from a rural, traditional past and thus in need of culturally sensitive medical development. To meet this perceived need, health care workers interpreted medicinal plants as objects that have scientific names as well as active ingredients, that must be prescribed by doctors rather than recommended by relatives or friends, and that are packaged in capsules, bottles, and tubes accompanied by instructions for use. By extending the set of social practices associated with biomedicine to popular medicine, the Farmácia Viva program effectively redeployed popular medicine as part of Fortaleza's hegemonic biomedical industry.

The pharmaceuticalizing process bears a certain similarity to some of the practices advocated by the doctor leading the health council meetings. As in that case, here Dr. Santos linked the achievement of good health to the understanding and undertaking of normative biomedical practices, which are themselves part and parcel of the neoliberal forms of governance pervasive in western market-driven democracies (Rose 2007). Although Dr. Santos's assessment of favela life was more sentimental, health care professionals in both situations perceived that residents' health depended on adjusting their expectations of what medical care actually is and becoming educated about how to access it appropriately.

Residents of Pirambu come equipped on all of these occasions with their own understandings of health, appropriate medical care, and good medicine. Farmácia Viva's traditional medical clinics were not particularly popular within the favela, but neither were they as widely scorned as has been reported in other parts of the world (Ugalde 1985; Van der Geest, Speckman, and Streefland 1990). Rather, residents viewed the clinics and their products with a pragmatic eye as "something that was better than nothing at all," in the words of a woman who was leaving a Farmácia Viva clinic.

CHAPTER FIVE

Favors, Rights, and the Management of Illness

In January 2003 then secretary of health for the state of Ceará Jurandi Frutuoso gave a radio interview at the Universidade Federal do Ceará about the dramatic improvements in health care that the state had realized since the implementation of the Sistema Único de Saúde. In addition to greater accessibility and higher-quality medical care, Frutuoso noted that changes had occurred in the way people thought about health care. "Before," he said, "it [health care] was like a favor. Today people know that they have the right to good health care. If a medication is not in stock, they demand to know why. They're more involved in the system."

During the late 1990s and early 2000s, Ceará invested additional sums of money into its health care system in order to complete the transition from the older model of care to the SUS model, in which municipal health departments were the primary entities responsible for planning, managing, and administering most aspects of health care. The health care professionals I spoke with during this period tended to affirm the health secretary's assertion, saying that as much as they were trying to improve the quality of health care in the state, they were also trying to change people's concepts of what health care is. The health councils as well as a door-to-door preventive health care program that I will describe later were presented to me as, in part, furthering the ideological goal of changing the concept of health care to something that was thought of as a right of citizenship.

This chapter and the next are devoted to an examination of the discourses and practices that surround health-seeking behavior in Pirambu in order to assess whether and how health care, as a particular type of citizenship right, was in fact assimilated by low-income residents. One of the social processes I am particularly interested in exploring is how moral valuations of health care become embedded in the worldviews of Pirambu's residents and then transformed across generations (Muehlebach 2011). Do younger generations express a greater sense of entitlement to or preference for certain kinds of medical services than older residents in the favela do? How do the older generations remember the medical care they received in the interior of the state, and how do they interpret their current levels of access to health care?

The choices that residents of all ages in Pirambu make about medical care are largely overdetermined by economic constraints. Poor residents of the city rely primarily on the robust network of public neighborhood health clinics and public health workers who come through the city's low-income neighborhoods on a regular basis. In contrast, the privatized tier of Brazil's health care system, epitomized by Fortaleza's towering glass and steel medical complexes with imaging and diagnostic laboratories as well as its boutique private *consultórios* (doctors' offices), remains emphatically out of reach for the majority of the city's low-income residents.

However, over the years that I spent conducting fieldwork in Pirambu I became increasingly curious about a pattern I observed in the ways that older and younger residents of the favela sought out and talked about medical care. Broadly speaking, the older residents appeared to rely contentedly on an extensive system of public health clinics for their medical care, while the younger residents, particularly those who were ascending economically and socially, complained bitterly about the public health care system and sought private medical care whenever they could. Valuations of and choices about medical services and technologies thus appeared to be deeply embedded in the subtle class and generational hierarchies of the favela. In this chapter I focus broadly on the experiences with medical care of what I refer to as the older generation of Pirambu and on the way those residents negotiate medical decisions for themselves and their family members. I attempt to understand how older residents' participation in the labor market and in political activism shaped their current understanding and practice of medical care as well as to examine the range of social practices that were necessary for residents to receive health care.

Generational Tension in the Favela

To call attention to a particular generation within Pirambu and to describe its social practices and discourses is complicated by the demographic situation that many people still live with their parents, grand-parents, uncles, and aunts long into adulthood, almost always until they marry and often longer. Moving out and establishing one's own home is itself a social aspiration achieved only by better-off favela residents. Thus when I was doing interviews regarding medical decision making and following examples of particular illness cases, I was confronted by several generations within one household and often heard multiple, con-tradictory answers to the questions I asked about healing and the health care system. Over time, I was able to discern a distinct pattern that di-vided elder residents' practices and discourses from those of the younger generation, and I then began to investigate it more deliberately.[1]

When I elicited accounts of illness experiences in Pirambu, I found that men and women who were over approximately fifty years of age and had been born in the interior were noticeably more enthusiastic about the network of public health clinics in the favela than their younger sib-lings and their children were. The older residents often favorably com-pared the care they received in Fortaleza to the stark absence of medical care they experienced growing up in the interior, and they would as-sert that access to medicine was in fact one of the primary reasons they moved to the capital city.

I also noticed that older residents rarely complained about the medi-cal care they received. Or if they happened to mention, for example, the long wait periods they endured at local medical clinics, they did so flatly, without providing an accompanying moral evaluation of that experi-ence. Finally, their narratives of obtaining health care often highlighted the favors they needed to procure that care, but they did not seem to in-terpret those favors as a contradiction to their putative right to care.

These were the same residents who when I collected their life histo-ries could remember Pirambu before it became a community with an extensive set of services and infrastructure. I was told what favela life was like when there was no or only minimally available electricity, flush toilets were nonexistent, and public transportation was not as regular or as convenient. Some of these residents either remembered participating themselves or were told about their parents' participation in the social protests of the 1950s, 1960s, and 1970s for the extension of rights and services to the favela.

As discussed earlier, the 1988 constitution was the culmination of a considerable broadening in the number of rights and the idea of citizen-ship in Brazil as initially set out in the 1934 constitution. Sweeping la-bor rights, including the right to a minimum wage, paid maternity and paternity leave, and retirement and health care benefits were just some of the gains enshrined in the 1988 constitution. The contemporary era in which I conducted fieldwork was largely perceived as "simpático" (kind or generous) by older residents of Pirambu despite their ongoing sense of exclusion from many of society's resources. Nonetheless, I observed older residents of Pirambu making only occasional use of notions of rights, justice, and citizenship in their daily lives and rarely putting forward claims to health care in these terms. When they did use such terms, the language showed up in unexpected contexts and sometimes was associated with surprising meanings. The following illness narrative helps to illustrate these points.

End of Life Care and Treatment

Fátima Vieira da Conceição was born in 1951 in Pecém, then a sleepy, rural, beach town on the Atlantic coast seventy miles northwest of Fortaleza and now with one of the largest ports in Ceará. When she was nine her father, a farmer and the sole breadwinner of the family, passed away. Shortly after his death Fátima's mother removed her from school and urged her to stay home, making and selling clothes to help support the family. When Fátima was twelve she was sent to Fortaleza to work as a live-in maid. Over a period of thirteen years she worked for five different families, sending the earnings home to her family in Pecém.

In 1976, at the age of twenty-five, Fátima met Raimundo, a heavy-drinking, alternately abusive and neglectful, older man. Raimundo had a wife and family, but over the next ten years Fátima gave birth to six of his children. While raising her children she worked making clothes in a factory near downtown Fortaleza and moved from one rented house to the next in different neighborhoods throughout the city. She was careful to point out to me that unlike the time when she had worked as a maid, her factory job was salaried, and she received health care and retirement benefits. "I finally had *bom trabalho* [good work], a job where I could support myself, something I had been looking for since I moved from the *interior*," she told me.

In 1986 Fátima heard from her younger sister Rafaela, who also moved to the city as a teenager, that a piece of land had been abandoned in Pirambu and if she acted quickly she might be able to claim a piece of it. With the help of her sister and a few friends Fátima built her first house from scraps of paper and cardboard, on the northern edge of Pirambu. During the twelve years that followed, Fátima continued to work at the clothing factory, gave birth to three more children, and slowly transformed her home into a sturdier construction of adobe and brick. Her work at the factory allowed her to maintain a relatively stable existence in the favela and provide for herself and her children with the help of the rare visit or gift from Raimundo and Rafaela, who was beginning to flourish in a neighborhood several miles west of Pirambu.

In October 1997 Fátima was diagnosed with cervical cancer. In recounting the story of her initial diagnosis she told me she had been feeling ill with abdominal pain for some time and had spoken about it with a neighbor who then went with her to the local health unit to get some relief for it. The nurse there felt a swelling in Fátima's abdomen and sent her to a larger clinic about a mile away for further testing. Fátima recounted that she had to go three days in a row, waking up early each morning for the chance of seeing a doctor there. Her oldest son knew a janitor at the clinic, and she ended up asking her son to request that the janitor hold a place in line for her. The doctor there gave her a referral for an appointment at the Instituto do Câncer do Ceará, a public hospital in Fortaleza dedicated entirely to the treatment and care of cancer patients. Fátima recalled that she was seen within the month at the hospital but that it was another three months until she received the test results confirming that she had cervical cancer. "It would have been longer," she commented, "but my sister's husband had a friend who worked in a pharmacy, and he was able to call and get them for me."

The doctors at the Instituto do Câncer suggested a complete hysterectomy immediately following the diagnosis, and she had the operation in April 1998. I asked her how she decided to go ahead with the operation and if she'd had any qualms about it. "There was no question for me," she replied. "It was totally paid for by the state, and it was what was indicated. My family needed me." I asked if she was surprised that such a big operation would be fully paid for. "No," she replied, "I've worked all my life. I've been a good worker. This is what a big city like Fortaleza can provide. It's so much better than the *interior*."

She told me that for six months following the operation she felt much better. Although she wasn't able to return to work, she helped her oldest son cover their living room floor with cement and managed to visit her sister's family occasionally as well. However, by the time I met her in October 1998 she was feeling ill again and expressed concern about the possibility of the cancer returning. "I can tell it's come back," Fátima said one day when a neighbor and I stopped by for a visit. "I didn't think they could take it away so easily."

"You should go back to the hospital," the neighbor urged her. "They'll be able to tell what's wrong."

Fátima shrugged her shoulders and said, "I'm through with that. Why should I go, just to hear them say I'm sick? I'm sick! I'm very sick." But the neighbor wouldn't give up so easily, and she eventually persuaded Fátima to speak with the nurse at the neighborhood health clinic. The nurse suggested that Fátima return to the medical clinic where her initial blood tests were done. And she did, again relying on the friend of her son to secure a place in line for her. The results of those tests, which arrived the following month, confirmed that the cancer had returned and had since spread throughout her body. Now the doctor at the Instituto do Câncer recommended chemotherapy, which would also be provided free of charge.

Initially, Fátima was reluctant to undergo the treatment. In addition to being wary of the effects involved, she expressed doubt about getting to the hospital, which was several long bus rides from her house, and about leaving her younger children on their own for extended periods. Meanwhile, her sister Rafaela had been on the phone with Fátima trying to persuade her to consider a private hospital for treatment. "She said she'd ask her co-worker about other options," Fátima told me. "She doesn't trust the doctors at the public hospital, and she thinks I'm not getting good care." I asked her what she thought. "To me it's all the same," she replied. "I just don't think I can go through with it at all. I don't have the resources for it."

Now several other neighbors got involved and pooled their money to enable Fátima to take the bus to the hospital. They also offered to look after her children for the days she was receiving treatment. I overheard one of her closer friends and neighbors, Mariana, tell her, "You've worked hard all of your life, you should be permitted this, you shouldn't die without care."

Fátima finally agreed to go, and I ended up going to the first appointment with her along with her neighbor Mariana. The Instituto do Câncer is in a vast complex of buildings that also houses Ceará's medical school as well as several other smaller hospitals and a breast-milk bank. Navigating the maze of buildings wasn't easy, but Mariana took the lead, completely undaunted, while Fátima hung back, enveloped and overwhelmed by the complex. The hospital waiting room was strikingly new, with plush, deep chairs, shiny television sets, and a large, well-tiled bathroom.

As we waited for Fátima's treatment to begin, Mariana told me something about herself. She was older than Fátima by nearly ten years and moved to Fortaleza in the early 1950s. Unlike Fátima, she remembered some of the social protests that took place in Pirambu in the late 1950s. "We took all of our concerns to the street then," she said. "We made sure the politicians knew what we wanted." She told me she had held only one salaried job in her life, making do the rest of the time with whatever informal labor she could find in the favela, but she hoped her children would find better employment, something that would come with benefits. I asked her what kind of benefits she thought were useful, given that health care was now free, as it was for Fátima. She responded that it was true, now they had the right to health care, but it took extra work for people to ensure that they got what they needed. When I asked what kind of work she was thinking of, she responded, "Sometimes you need a favor in order to secure your rights."

Her observation came back to me as we were leaving the hospital that evening and a nurse recommended a medication that would help ease Fátima's pain. The nurse said Fátima could pick up the medication for free at the hospital's pharmacy, but Mariana thought this was unlikely, given how often public pharmacies ran out of stock. Mariana suggested that we contact her aunt who worked at one of the pharmacies in Fortaleza and might be able to get the medication at a discount. The line for the pharmacy was long as we were leaving, and Mariana said she'd call her aunt that evening. Several days later Mariana returned to Fátima's house with the sought-after medication.

Mariana continued to help Fátima through the biweekly treatments, rounding up neighbors to help pay for her transportation and look after her children. She also called a cousin who was able to talk to a nurse at the Instituto do Câncer to change Fatima's biweekly appointments to a day that fit better with her children's school schedule. But eventually Fátima decided to stop attending the chemotherapy sessions.

I ran into her youngest son, William, then ten years old, the week after her decision to stop treatment, and I accompanied him back to his house, where I found Fátima lying bedridden in a hammock, thin as a rail, and now completely bald from the chemotherapy treatments. Fátima explained that the treatment had become too much to bear. "Having to worry about the money and who would watch William and the others—I couldn't take it. My relationship with my sister is too weak, and I don't know enough people here in the favela," she said as she gestured to her surroundings. In the final days before she died, her extended family gathered at her house day and night. Although they seemed reconciled to her death, her sister Rafaela continued to hold that if they had gotten Fátima to a "good hospital" they could have at least prolonged her life.

Fátima died on June 6, 1999, a little over five months after she was told the cancer had returned and spread. Her funeral was a dispirited affair held at a public gravesite some ways outside of Fortaleza, both emphasizing Fátima's powerlessness as a poor favela dweller and causing further anguish for her family. A week later I attended a seventh-day mass for Fátima that another friend arranged. The service was held at one of the larger Catholic churches in Pirambu to ask blessings for Fátima and the two other residents who died the week before. Eight of Fátima's nine children attended the mass; they stood neatly dressed in freshly washed clothes, visibly distraught by their mother's death.

Working for Health

In Fátima's case, her neighbor Mariana made an illuminating comment with regard to the continued necessity of favors to facilitate favela life. Many of the older residents in Pirambu could remember a time when health care and other important services could only be obtained through favors. Isabella, the woman I lived with during my first period of fieldwork, often remarked that when she lived in the interior she had to make a trip to see the mayor's wife and promise support for her husband in the next election in order to get basic pharmaceuticals at a discount. Residents like Isabella and Fátima, like most older residents of Pirambu, had moved from small towns and rural areas of Ceará that were dominated by feudalism and other forms of paternalistic social relationships. In these places poor families often depended upon the heads of more affluent households for whom they worked not only for wages but also for gifts and favors they bestowed over the course of their relationships (Scheper-Hughes 1992). Fátima had recalled that after her father died, her mother began doing the washing for a wealthier woman in their small village who generously supplied the family with baskets of fruits and vegetables, occasional meat, and payment for medical bills. When Fátima moved to Fortaleza and began working as a maid for families in the city, she hoped for a similar kind of "*amizade*" (friendship) with her employers, she said. But only one of her *patrões* (bosses) was "truly good" and gave her bonuses to send home to her family.

Part of the aim of the 1988 constitution, with its attention to civil rights and the rights of minorities, was specifically to erode these paternalistic relationships and to put in their place the knowledge that services such as health care were rights of citizenship, not favors bestowed by wealthy patrons. The narrative of Fátima's illness points to some of the obstacles that might prevent residents of Pirambu from recognizing health care as such a right. Fátima knew that the state was responsible for paying for her hysterectomy, and she was quick to justify its being performed free of charge by stating that she had worked all her life and furthermore had been a good worker. Here Fátima conceptualized her right to health care as deriving from specific moral and social categories. This is what James Holston has called "special treatment rights," that is, rights that are bestowed on particular categories of citizens, such as factory workers (Holston 2008). Thus although Fátima recognized on some level that health care is a right, she did not have in mind the form that the constitution advocates, in which entitlements like health care are linked to Brazilian citizenship in general. Rather, residents like Fátima who actually held jobs in the formal economy learned to link health benefits to salaried work. This was symbolically affirmed every time they presented their social security cards as proof of employment in the formal labor market, even after doing so no longer was required, in exchange for health care services.

The 1988 constitution formally dissolved the link between labor and health care and instead tied health care services to one's status as a citizen of Brazil. The reforms made medical care vastly more accessible to low-income citizens throughout Brazil (Paim et al. 2011), in part by doing away with the requirement of presenting documentation such as a social security card before receiving care. Despite these changes, older residents of Pirambu who had worked in the formal economy or had relatives or close friends with such experience tended to associate the availability of health care with their participation in the labor market rather than the beneficence of the Brazilian state. An example provided in the next narrative demonstrates that this association of health care with work was evident not only at the level of discourse but also of practice, as some older residents adhered habitually to outdated routines such as presenting their social security cards at medical appointments.

Among the many residents who had no contact with the formal labor market, I found that the experience of free health care benefits was most often attributed to the fact of living in Fortaleza rather than the *interior*. I remember a conversation at a public clinic in the city between an older resident named Alícia and another woman. Alícia took her daughter to the clinic and fell into conversation with the other woman, who had come from the *interior* and was evidently worried about how she would pay for her visit. "I was told to come to the city because the doctors are better here, but I'm not sure how we'll manage the cost," she told Alícia. "Well, you're right about that," Alícia acknowledged. "The *interior* has nothing, I remember that. But when you live in the city, it's free."

Throughout my fieldwork I saw a pattern repeated in almost all of the medical histories I collected from older residents in the favela. These residents consistently presented negative evaluations of medical care in the *interior* and often referred to it as "muito fraco" (very weak). "The medical system in the *interior* is weak?" I'd ask. "No, no, the medicine—the medicine is weak there" would come the reply. These accounts were followed by lengthy examples of residents' increased access to medical care once they had moved to Fortaleza and how much stronger pharmaceuticals were than the "plantas medicinais" (traditional medicines) they had used in the *interior*.

When I asked residents to describe particular medical events I was often provided with accounts of prolonged, futile encounters with the medical system in Fortaleza, but these encounters were routinely regarded as successful by the residents themselves; these narratives were typically grounded in comparisons with their experiences in the *interior* and decorated with gratitude at receiving any medical attention at all. Thus, the experience of medical care and the luxury of not having to pay for it were attributed by older residents either to their participation in the formal labor market, however brief, or to the mere fact of having moved from rural, poverty-stricken areas to a flourishing city. I rarely heard any older residents mention the 1988 constitution or the shift in entitlements that accompanied it.

The Mota Vaz Family

When I started my fieldwork in 1998, one of my first extensive interviews on illness and medical treatment in Pirambu was with Maria Clara Mota Vaz. She moved to Pirambu from a small town in 1993, and I thought she would be able to give me a broad sense of how her expectations of health care and available treatment options changed upon moving to the city. When I told her I wanted to talk about access to medical care in the favela, she stopped me and asked, "You want to talk about health in Pirambu? Have I told you about Fernanda?" I shook my head. "Let me tell you what's happened to Fernanda, and then you will know something about medical care in Pirambu," she said. Fernanda was Maria Clara's nine-year-old granddaughter who came to live with her while the girl's mother, Solange, was working as a live-in *empregada* for a wealthy family in Fortaleza. "I just got back from taking Fernanda to the hospital this morning," Maria Clara said. "She doesn't eat well, and she's had attacks of vomiting, so my son and I took her to the hospital. And do you know what the doctor said?" Again I shook my head. "That she has the height and weight of a six-year-old! Fernanda's nine and a half." I asked her what treatment the doctor prescribed, and she replied, "He doesn't know yet. He's ordered a bunch of tests for her." And then she proceeded to enumerate them: "He took a blood test, urine samples, and made some X-rays of her hand, and he's going to send us to a specialist."

In order to see the specialist they would have to first go to the Centro de Diabetes e Hipertensão (Center for Diabetes and Hypertension) where the specialist worked to set up an appointment. The clinic was two bus rides away, and she didn't see how she was going to come up with that sort of money, about two dollars at the time. I offered to cover the bus fare, and Maria Clara gladly accepted and allowed as to how we should probably go the following morning.

At 6:30 the next morning Maria Clara and Fernanda stopped by on their way to the bus stop. Fernanda was dressed in a clean, neatly pressed party frock, her hair was carefully combed, and she proudly announced that she was missing school for the day. Her grandmother was dressed in a clean skirt and blouse. She was clearly anxious about the trip and clutched the directions to the clinic, Fernanda's blood test, and her own social security card tightly as the crowded morning bus lurched down the streets toward the city center.

When we finally got off the bus we quickly discovered that we were in the wrong place; the Center for Diabetes was at the other end of town. Disappointed by the day's turn of events, Maria Clara reasoned that it was too late to try to get there to make the appointment and that we might as well return to Pirambu. On the bus ride home Maria Clara commented that the early morning bus rides reminded her of when she used to work in the cashew-processing factory that loomed just blocks outside of Pirambu. "I worked there for ten years," she said. "I never got to know the city, but that's why I know the buses so well." It was just past nine in the morning when we finally made our way back down the alley to our respective homes.

Over the next week Maria Clara tried to persuade one of her sons who had connections to a doctor at the diabetes center to make an appointment with the specialist directly rather than have to appear in person to do so. She was eventually successful, and three weeks later we set out again for the city. This time we made it to the Center for Diabetes in under an hour and were sent to take a number and wait in line with about ten or twelve other patients and their family members. After waiting close to three hours on the skinny, wooden benches outside the clinic door, we were finally shown in to see an endocrinologist, Dr. Letícia Socorro. The doctor, a young woman of about thirty, asked Fernanda how she was and then weighed and measured her. She confirmed that Fernanda was the standard height and weight of a girl six rather than nine years old. Maria Clara brought out the now slightly worn X-rays of Fernanda's hands and her own social security card, which she handed to the doctor. "You don't need those any more," the doctor said, pushing the card back to her. "But I've worked for a long time, and I have my card from it," Maria Clara protested. "No, *senhora*, it's okay now. With the SUS we don't need to see that you worked or where you worked. It's enough that you're here."

Maria Clara looked dubious, but she tucked the card into her handbag and turned her attention back to the doctor. "Now," said the doctor, pointing to Fernanda, "you're her mother?" "Grandmother," Maria Clara corrected her, somewhat sheepishly. "Well then, we'll need to do another round of tests, a blood test, and more X-rays just to eliminate the possibility that something serious is wrong. But I think she might be lacking an important hormone."

Then she began to describe a government program that offered undersize children hormonal supplements. She explained that the program was funded by the state of Ceará and that if Fernanda qualified it would provide her with free growth hormones. The doctor said the program had been very successful so far, and they would just need to wait until there was room for Fernanda. She stated that she was sure Fernanda would be able to join the program by the new year, then some six months away.

Maria Clara asked the doctor if she was sure the hormones would be free. "Oh yes," replied the doctor, "you're to get everything for free. But until that time Fernanda should take vitamins." And she proceeded to fill out a prescription for vitamins.

As we left, there was a sigh of relief and elation from Maria Clara. She turned to me, smiling, and said, "It was worth it after all, all this waiting—a free government program and the hormones that we'll get for free. Solange will be very happy, won't she?"

Once we arrived back in Pirambu, Maria Clara quickly sought out her sister Isabel and began to tell her about the government program and the free hormone treatments that Fernanda would likely be receiving. She also mentioned she was going to call Solange, Fernanda's mother, and tell her about the treatments. Over the next few weeks I heard Maria Clara tell a number of her neighbors about the government hormone program in which Fernanda would soon be enrolled. The topic was generally brought up in a casual way, with a friend asking about how the three grandchildren who lived with Maria Clara were doing and Maria Clara replying that they were all fine but that Fernanda was particularly lucky because she had seen a doctor who was going to enroll her in a free *programa de hormônio*. If the friend or neighbor asked what a hormone program was, as they usually did, Maria Clara explained that Fernanda wasn't growing as she should and that she was "missing a hormone." The doctor they had seen offered to enroll Fernanda in a free government program that would give her medicine to replace the hormone she was missing. At this point most people pointed out that God must be on her side or that she had good luck to live in a *cidade bem rica* (a wealthy city) like Fortaleza, and the conversation moved on to other topics.

The discussion with Solange, however, apparently had not gone as smoothly. "Solange doesn't want me to enroll Fernanda in the program," Maria Clara told me one morning. "Why not?" I asked. "She thinks it won't be any good because it's a government health program, and she wants me to wait to bring her to see a private doctor in Aldeota [a higher-income neighborhood in Fortaleza]," replied Maria Clara. "She said that her boss might be able to get Fernanda an appointment with her doctor." There was a pause. "I don't know, though. I'm not sure we should wait. It seems like a fine program that the doctor told us about. She seemed very honest," Maria Clara said. Iterations of this dynamic continued throughout the remaining months of my first period of fieldwork. Maria Clara waited patiently and without comment for Fernanda's name to appear on the government-approved list for hormone growth supplements, while Solange pursued her own connections to obtain a private consultation for Fernanda with more evident frustration but an unequally uncertain outcome.

When I arrived back in Pirambu almost one year later, in the fall of 2000, to conduct follow-up fieldwork, one of my first visits was to Maria Clara's house. With considerable pride she showed me all of the renovations her home had undergone during the previous year. The formerly dirt floor was now covered in wide, tan tiles, a flush toilet had been installed, and a large refrigerator now sat in the tiny kitchen. "This is all due to Solange's boss," Maria Clara explained. "She's been lending her extra money to help pay for these improvements. She's very generous, a good woman."

I asked after Fernanda, and it was then that she told me Fernanda had grown hardly at all in the time that I had been gone. "She's now just a centimeter taller than she was before," she confided. Not only had Fernanda hardly grown, she still hadn't been put on the government-funded hormone-supplement program. Maria Clara said the doctor told her during their last visit six months earlier that she was "moving slowly up the list." They had another appointment at the same clinic at the end of the month, and Maria Clara asked me if I would be willing to go with them as I did the year before.

On the appointed morning I arrived at Maria Clara's house at the early hour of 6 a.m. Fernanda, nearly eleven now, showed all the signs of fast becoming a teenager. She was still concerned about what to wear to the hospital, but this year it was a variety of jeans rather than dresses that she was deciding among and a belt that she put on and took off, deliberating as to whether it complemented her outfit. Maria Clara was still the anxious, overworked grandmother of the year before. There was the usual flurry of excitement as she made sure she had all the documents she needed for the trip. The last item she took from her house was the Bible, in which she had carefully pressed the X-rays the doctor gave her almost a year and a half before.

As we made our way to the bus stop, Maria Clara explained that although having to wait so long to enter the government program was beginning to weigh on her, she was still confident that eventually Fernanda would receive the care she had been promised. Solange was still disparaging about the possibility that the government program would actually do Fernanda any good, but for now she had given up actively trying to dissuade her mother from pursuing it. And Maria Clara commented, "Solange works well with her boss. She's done so much for her, so maybe she'll be able to find a doctor for Fernanda too. But until then . . .," and here she trailed off as we ascended into the bus.

Informal Medical Practices and Generational Differences in the Favela

The narrative above as well as Fátima's earlier story urges us to consider not just how older residents interpret medical care but also the social practices necessary to obtain it. An explicit goal of the health care reforms laid out in the 1988 constitution was to enable those Brazilians without access to wealth, social connections, or political capital to obtain adequate health care. Although public medical clinics see patients free of charge and most services and medications are supposed to be provided for free, Maria Clara's pursuit of care for her granddaughter and Fátima's case, as well as dozens of other medical histories I collected and interviews I conducted throughout the favela, suggests that calling on social networks and connections remains an important tactic in obtaining health services and medicines. During the entire course of my fieldwork, I found that residents of Pirambu used their connections with family members, neighbors, friends, and acquaintances of higher social status at all stages in the process of attaining medical care, from making appointments, scheduling medical tests, and obtaining test results to interpreting doctor's diagnoses and purchasing pharmaceuticals.

I first became aware of this pattern when I noticed that residents engaged in rather extensive investments of time and social contacts to save money on medicines or simply to be able to purchase it in the first place. Although the state was mandated to provide a long list of medications for free, often they were not available when residents went to claim them. Even when they were available, I occasionally observed residents forgoing generic brands in order to avail themselves of more expensive name-brand pharmaceuticals at private pharmacies. In both instances, residents of Pirambu turned to their social networks to facilitate the purchases.

Fátima's case is a good example of this. At her friend Mariana's encouragement, she chose not to wait in line at the hospital's public pharmacy, where she might be able to obtain the medication she needed for free, and relied instead on Mariana to contact a relative of hers who worked at a pharmacy and thus might be able to get the medication at a discount.

I witnessed this tactic, in which state or market procedures to acquire medicines were circumvented by informal relations, employed re-peatedly throughout the favela without discrimination as to a resident's age, gender, or social status. However, as I describe in the next chap-ter, the ends to which this tactic was directed varied with respect to age. Older residents like Fátima and younger residents like Solange were equally able to get medications more cheaply or for free through fam-ily or friends working in the medical arena or through former or current bosses, or they had family members to lend or give them the money to purchase what they needed. What they rarely did was simply walk to the nearest pharmacy, public or private, and receive or purchase the medica-tions they needed themselves.

Residents of Pirambu invested in social networks to facilitate other interactions with the health care system as well, such as making doc-tors' appointments, obtaining test results, and avoiding waiting in line. Fátima's and Maria Clara's cases illustrate this point. Fátima's initial ap-pointment after seeing a nurse at the health clinic required her to wait in a very long line to see a doctor at the public clinic. Through her son's friend she was able to hold a place in line so she did not have to spend the entire day there herself. Fátima also called upon her social connec-tions to facilitate delivery of her test results; she waited three months without hearing from the doctor, at which point one of her children suggested she call the hospital. Fátima professed to being too intimi-dated to call the hospital herself, so she asked her younger sister to call for her. Her sister's husband worked in a pharmaceutical laboratory and asked a colleague of his to make the phone call to ask that the results be sent immediately. Shortly thereafter, Fátima received the diagnosis that she had cancer.

Maria Clara appeared less dependent on her social relationships to facilitate the medical appointments for Fernanda, although she did have her son put in a call to the Center for Diabetes to schedule an appoint-ment for Fernanda. A more surprising aspect of Maria Clara's narrative was the disjuncture between her own and her daughter Solange's valua-tion of the diagnosis and proposed treatment for Fernanda. Maria Clara used her social relationship with her son to facilitate access to a public medical good, the government-sponsored growth-hormone treatment protocol. Her attitude remained relatively positive throughout a nearly two-year delay for Fernanda's name simply to come off the waiting list for the program, entailing lengthy bus rides, early morning risings, and hours and hours outside of doctors' offices.

Solange, on the other hand, immediately rejected the proposed treatment as being ineffective specifically because it was a government program. She sought to use her own social connections toward the pursuit of private rather than public health care for her daughter. Although it became clear the following year that Solange had successfully negotiated some assistance from the family for whom she worked, it had come in the form of housing improvements rather than medical resources. From Maria Clara's perspective, this tradeoff was intelligible; patronage was sorely needed for expensive commodities such as floor tiles, but medical care was something she could seek in a public realm and that she appeared to consider at least sufficient if not commensurate with private care.

Maria Clara did not participate in the social activism that galvanized the community of Pirambu in the 1940s and 1950s, as she only arrived later, in the 1980s, but she had certainly heard about it from her close family and neighbors, how it was ignited by vehement opposition to the inequalities of life in the favela. But the opposition seemed to soften somewhat for the older generation, as expressed, for example, in the presumption of relative equality in health care services. On the other hand, Solange's censure of the government-run health care program that her mother sought for Fernanda could indicate that this view has not extended across generations. Rather, for some younger residents of the favela a growing frustration with inequality is emerging alongside an individualism that views social relationships and networks as a way to attain privatized rather than public forms of health care.

Recent ethnographies of medical practice around the world have drawn attention to the pervasiveness of informal networks and reciprocal relations of favors as a means of obtaining scarce medical goods and services (Andaya 2009, Béhague 2002, Brotherton 2012, Salmi 2003). What makes their continued use in Pirambu striking is that Brazil's formal health care ideology since 1988 has been predicated on the twin ideas that health care is a human right and that it is the duty of the state to provide basic health care services. In keeping with these ideals, city officials in Fortaleza have invested in public health programs that aim in part to strengthen low-income residents' relationship with the state and to decrease their reliance on informal networks of care. Nonetheless, social mediation persists in Pirambu at virtually every point in the process of seeking medical care. These tactics were rarely criticized by older residents and, as I discuss below, were instead viewed as accepted means to an end—*a dar um jeito* (to find a way), to use social influence to circumvent obstacles—to manage the exigencies of daily life in the favela.

Juridicalizing Health

Despite the seeming remarkableness of the medical care that Fátima and Fernanda received—that they received care at all and largely at no cost to themselves—from an outsider's perspective there were several discouraging aspects of their care. Perhaps most alarmingly, Fátima was made to wait three-plus months for test results that if provided earlier might have saved or prolonged her life. Although rarely this consequential, instances of waiting prolonged periods for health care appointments and treatments were common for residents of Pirambu, as was having to pay for one's own pharmaceuticals because the state pharmacy was out of stock.

New scholarship has investigated the possibility that courts might provide an alternative institutionalized voice for the poor to allow them to realize their right to health care through civil rights litigation (Biehl and Petryna 2011; Ferraz 2009, 2011). Lawsuits have been filed for a wide range of treatments but are increasing particularly rapidly for prescribed pharmaceuticals in states throughout Brazil (Biehl et al. 2012). As yet, however, there is no evidence that this practice is perceived as a viable possibility for favela residents in Fortaleza who receive inadequate medical treatment or drugs.

Low-income residents, old and young, continue to lack confidence in the civil sphere of their society that might otherwise offer an opportunity to protect their rights under the constitution. I witnessed countless examples of this phenomenon in Pirambu throughout the years I conducted fieldwork. For example, despite the constitution's strict regulations regarding the number of hours of work permitted per week, employers in Fortaleza flagrantly violated them. This practice was totally normalized, and residents I knew suffered the indignities without ever contemplating the possibility of taking their employers to court.

Likewise, I never observed residents in the favela discuss the possibility of going to court for the right to access services or medications. If residents of Fortaleza were demanding more from the public health care system, as the city secretary of health asserted, they were not the older residents I knew in Pirambu. This can be attributed to many of the causes already discussed, including elderly residents' tendency to associate health benefits with employment rather than citizenship, their distrust of the legal system, and their reluctance to find fault with the little injustices associated with the health care they do receive. Thus while some broad presumptions of equality and access to health care appear to have been woven into older residents' perspectives, I saw no evidence that the idea of health care as a right was something that could be claimed in court. Health care workers in the community actually remarked upon residents' passivity. I remember talking to a family health care assistant about the challenges that older favela residents face seeking health care. She commented, "People have to get up so early here just to go stand in line, and even then they don't know for sure if they will get help. But they just say '*Se Deus quiser*' (If God wills it) as though it's normal and there's nothing they can do about it."

Indeed, older residents rarely offered a moral commentary on the difficulties they experienced in the public health care system. Unlike younger residents in the favela who commented at length about the inadequacies and indignities of public health care, their elders often reframed the problems they experienced as being the result of inadequate social networks. Fátima was deeply concerned about how to pay for transportation to and from the hospital where she was to receive treatment and how to manage care for her children and household while she was gone. She successfully mobilized friends, neighbors, and family members to help her address these issues but eventually was overwhelmed and attributed her unwillingness to continue with treatment to these dilemmas. Her final remarks here were telling, that she did not have a strong relationship with her sister and did not know enough people in the favela. Thus she offered a moral commentary not on the state of public health for the poor in Fortaleza but on her relationships with her sister and fellow residents of the favela.

In general, investing in associations with friends, neighbors, and acquaintances around matters of health was perceived by older residents of Pirambu not as currying favor or exploiting opportunities but rather as engaging (or not) in what were largely unremarked-upon acts of *dividindo* (sharing medical and other consumer goods), *carinho* (bestowing extra affection and care upon the ill and their family members), and *ajuda* (offering help, assistance, support, and relief in times of need).[2] From an outsider's perspective these acts may recall Michel de Certeau's descriptions of the survival practices of the poor, in which in the absence of any real power, an act "must play on and with a terrain imposed on it" to take advantage of opportunities to manage daily struggles (quoted in Scheper-Hughes 1992, 472), while from the perspective of older favela residents an act of survival was regarded instead as part of ongoing and long-standing practices of reciprocity in the favela. As with the residents of the shantytown Scheper-Hughes describes in her ethnography *Death without Weeping*, such tactics help to ameliorate and temporarily reshape situations. But unlike the social protests of previous decades in Pirambu, they do not ultimately challenge the broader political and economic contexts in which they occur.

CHAPTER SIX

Public and Private Medical Care
for a New Generation in Pirambu

As my research in Pirambu expanded, I began to observe more and more of the younger residents I knew in the favela pursuing private medical care and insurance in addition to the public care they consumed for free. Although there is broad concern about the growth of private health care in Brazil, the consumption of private care by low-income residents has received scant attention.[1] An article in the medical journal *The Lancet* highlights the challenges that growth in private medical care and insurance have posed for Brazil's public health care system (Paim et al. 2011). The authors focus attention on the growth of private medical care and insurance among the middle and upper-middle classes, making the assumption that it was too expensive for working-class or poor Brazilians to obtain.

Indeed, the purchase of private medical care and insurance is expensive; nonetheless, some residents of the favela, particularly the younger ones, have pursued it with a doggedness I previously associated only with the goals of higher education and fixed wage employment. I noticed, for example, that although younger residents still relied on the public system, they were far more likely than older residents to remark disapprovingly on their experience of it—the long waits they had to endure, the relative ineptness of the doctors, and the lack of dignity with which they were treated.

In my conversations with a small group of younger residents and their friends and family members it became apparent that they were consuming status and a sense of upward mobility as they consumed health care and that the choices they made about medical care were an embodiment of a broader phenomenon: the emergence of a consumer-oriented subjectivity in the favela. My interviews and experiences with younger residents suggest, as others have argued, that among at least some of the young, urban poor in Northeastern Brazil, consumption has become the primary means to enhance and capitalize on one's subjectivity and increasingly citizenship itself is being defined in terms of the ability to realize individual choice and self-enhancement (Edmonds 2007, O'Dougherty 2002, Rose 1999). In the following narrative I explore this developing subjectivity through the lens of medical decision making and suggest that paradoxically the universal right to health care guaranteed by the constitution goes unclaimed by a new generation of young favela residents for whom health care appears to be neither a favor nor a right but rather something that, in its privatized form, has become an aspiration.

The Lima Family

I first became alerted to the sharp distinction that younger residents in the favela drew between public and private medical care when, during my first period of fieldwork I was discussing the prevalence of children with asthma in Pirambu with a young family I had just met. Edson and Staci were unusual in that they had only one child, Ana, and did not want to have more. With just one child the parents could afford to invest all of their resources, dreams, and not insignificant worries into Ana. One of the most noticeable ways that this attention manifested was in the choices Edson and Staci made about Ana's medical care. Although younger residents of Pirambu like Edson and Staci often made use of public health clinics in their neighborhood, they expressed much more concern about doing so than residents of their parents' generation did. They were also much more likely to put their economic and social resources toward the purchase of private medical care and treatments. The following narrative offers an opportunity to examine these practices.

Edson Lima and his wife, Staci, belonged to that small but growing number of young favela residents with high aspirations. Edson was born in the interior in 1968 and moved to Fortaleza as a young boy. Staci was born in a neighborhood near Pirambu in 1975, and the couple met through friends in 1990. They lived in the heart of Pirambu in a well-kept, two-bedroom house. Though it was small the house had certain features that distinguished it from other homes in the neighborhood and pointed to its owners' middle-class ambitions. First, the Limas owned their home rather than renting it. About a quarter of the residents in Pirambu were homeowners; the others rented from landlords or were new to the area and taking over vacant land by squatting on it and constructing temporary homes of cardboard and wood. Edson was in the fortunate quarter of the population that managed to become homeowners, and he bought his house for about two thousand reais (approximately nine hundred dollars in 1997). He explained that he and his wife had saved money for almost five years and then received a gift of one thousand reais from a wealthy Fortaleza man Edson befriended while the man was doing charity work in the favela.

The house was the couple's tangible evidence that they were destined to realize some of their ambitious goals, and they made improvements to it whenever they could. Glazed cement covered the floor rather than unfinished cement or dirt. There was a separate bedroom that Edson and Staci shared, and they slept on a double bed rather than in hammocks, which were conventional bedding in rural Brazil. The house had a rather large indoor bathroom with bright-green tile on the floor and a toilet. All of these details, combined with Edson's steady job as a janitor at an English-language institute (Instituto Brazil–Estados Unidos, IBEU) in the city that paid nearly three times the going minimum wage, were enough to set the family apart from many of their friends and neighbors.

My discussions with Edson focused primarily on his hopes for his daughter, her future, and the day that she would be able to attend a private grammar school or the city university. It was Staci who was more focused on the daily details of Ana's well-being, including her health. When I first spent the afternoon with Staci, she said that if she had her choice she would stay home every day with her daughter and look after her. But even with Edson's relatively good pay she had to work to make ends meet every month. Staci worked four days a week selling bikinis in a small boutique on the other side of the city. She also took a computer class on Monday and Thursday evenings that she was able to attend for free because a brother of a friend of hers worked there. She was learning the Windows 95 operating system and a couple of application programs with the hope that this knowledge would enable her to find a job that was better than the one she currently had. She explained that even if she were still to work in the service industry she would need computer skills because even for these jobs employers were starting to prefer workers who had at least minimal computer knowledge.

Staci complained that one of the biggest disadvantages of working was that Ana seemed to get sick more often while she was away. Ana had come down with a cold and, like other children I observed in the favela, was diagnosed with asthma.[2] Two days before our conversation, Staci took her to a doctor, and she had to stay overnight at the hospital. Staci described the conditions there: "We took her to a public hospital, so she was forced to share a room with other patients. The hospital was dirty, like most public hospitals are. It almost was more dangerous to leave her there than it would have been to not go to the hospital altogether." A few minutes later she commented that the next time they went to a hospital it was going to be to a private one recommended to Edson by one of his co-workers.

I asked her what she thought the difference was between public and private hospitals in Fortaleza, and she responded immediately, "Oh there's a big difference. You can't trust public hospitals here at all, the ones the SUS sends you to. You have to go to the private ones to get good service." I pressed on: Did she think public hospitals in general had a reputation for being dangerous, or were she and Edson more cautious than other residents? She paused to reflect and then responded, "Everyone knows this, to be treated well, with dignity, this only happens at private hospitals. There they treat you like an individual, they really listen to you. I think my mother, for example, she doesn't notice this as much. She's used to waiting, so she doesn't mind the public clinics."

Another advantage of Edson's job was that initially it offered the family health insurance. Staci said that when Edson first started working for IBEU all three of them, Edson, Ana, and herself, had health insurance through IBEU. "We were very excited about this. We didn't know anyone else who could obtain private insurance through their job. And I told you, the public hospitals you see through the SUS are terrible. But," she continued, "it was too expensive, so we stopped it. Now we only have health insurance for Ana because if something were to happen to her, we would worry unless she had insurance." At thirty-eight reais a month, the insurance premium was a luxury that no other families I knew in Pirambu could afford.

As she began to swing Ana in the hammock, I noticed several bottles of cough medication on the large TV set that dominated the room. Among them was a bottle of *lambedor para tosse* (cough syrup) produced by Farmácia Viva. I asked Staci where she got it and if she had tried it yet. She told me one of the doctors at the local clinic had some extra bottles around that Farmácia Viva passed out to promote its program.

"He gave them to me for free, so of course I accepted them," she said. "But I don't like to use the *medicina popular* (folk medicine) too much, not for Ana. It's much better when we get pharmaceuticals like this," and she held up an unopened bottle of Tylenol. "Edson's co-workers or students sometimes give us medications, and that's where we get the good things."

I pressed Staci on what she meant by her comment that folk medicine wasn't for Ana. Farmácia Viva made an effort to target young mothers and their children, so if the medications it produced weren't for Ana, who were they for? Staci appeared exasperated by the question. "Ana deserves better than that," she responded. "We always try to give her the best, the best medicine, the best education, the best food. I even feel badly sometimes that we live here. If we didn't live here, in the favela, she wouldn't be sick. It's the dirty air that makes her lungs sick. As soon as Edson can save up enough money to buy a house, we're going to try to move closer to town, to one of the better neighborhoods."

Emerging Communities

Staci and Edson were more focused, better educated, and more self-conscious and articulate about their goals than many of the residents I knew in Pirambu, but they were certainly not alone in their accomplishments and aspirations. Teresa Caldeira has observed of the peripheral areas of São Paulo that "although the symbol of the periphery tends to homogenize, the conditions of life in the peripheral areas of the city are far from homogeneous" (2006, 115).

The residents I am discussing here were part of a small but growing minority that I observed in Pirambu who perceived themselves to be a cut above the average favela dweller and yearned for a "vida mais rica" (a richer life). They were young, they tended to have been born in Fortaleza rather than the interior, and they ardently believed in the dream of social mobility. As in the case of Staci and Edson, these residents also tended to express their aspirations for private medical care in terms of a broader desire to accomplish more than their parents had and perhaps eventually to move out of the favela altogether. *Medicina pública* (public medicine) was thought to be, as Staci put it, dirty and dangerous and to involve long waits to see doctors with inferior skills. For these younger residents, public health care tended to be associated with the poor-quality services of the rural interior or was an example of *a pior cara de favela* (the worst aspect or face of a favela). *Medicina particular* (private medicine), on the other hand, was thought to provide individualized care by doctors who were well educated and above all to treat even residents from the favela with dignity.

I observed this preference for private medical care in cases that required complex medical treatment as well as those that required minimal attention. A young married woman I knew, Vanessa, suffered a stroke one afternoon, and with a swollen tongue and her face half-paralyzed was taken immediately to a nearby public health clinic by her aunt. Vanessa, in her account to me of her health experience, emphasized that she had only gone to the public clinic because her family did not have private medical insurance, so this was all she could do. At the clinic, she spoke with a doctor who told her she was likely to have a brain tumor and that she was going to die. She confided, however, that this assessment didn't really worry her, as she knew that the doctors in the public hospitals were "terrible." She added, "They're all like this, they will just say anything to get you out the door more quickly. They're not as good as the educated ones are in the private hospitals." The doctor at the public clinic told her she had to complete a variety of tests to find out if she had actually had a stroke or if there was some other problem. Before she went back for tests, though, Vanessa and her husband called a prosperous cousin of hers who lived in the Aldeota neighborhood. "I was hoping he could get us in to see a private doctor. I needed an MRI exam," she said, "and if we waited to get one through the public system—forget it! It would have taken two years. You just have to find a way to get around the system." Vanessa's cousin eventually agreed to pay for a consultation at a private medical clinic, where the doctors confirmed the initial diagnosis of a stroke.

The preference for private medical care among the younger generation in Pirambu was also notable in much less severe cases of ill health. A young woman's nephew Pedro took a bad fall and knocked one of his upper teeth loose. His aunt Francine took him to the small clinic inside the Sindicato dos Trabalhadores dos Guias de Turismo do Ceará (Labor Union of Tour Guides of Ceará), where she worked as a secretary. Although the clinic technically was part of the SUS, patients had to work for the labor union or be a member of the union to be treated there. Francine allowed that the clinic staff also saw family members of those who were on good terms with the labor union's boss. After an hour or so of waiting in line at the clinic, Pedro was told that he could either have a root canal or have his tooth pulled. Both options were free, and the clinic itself was around the corner from Francine's house in Pirambu. Nonetheless, when I spoke with her that evening, Francine confided that she persuaded her mother to divert some money they generally saved for church tithing to pay for private dental care in Fortaleza. "He'll get much better treatment there, Jessica," Francine said. "And the dentist in the clinic at the *sindicato*, he didn't even treat us like people. He was so disrespectful!" When I asked her what she meant by disrespectful, she replied, "He just came in and asked me what happened without even really looking at me. He never asked Pedro anything, and he didn't even look at the tooth."

To avoid the public health care system, younger residents of Pirambu purchased single appointments with private health care providers, as was done in the cases described above, or they could purchase private health insurance plans that allowed them to see a range of providers for covered services. Private insurance plans were extremely rare in the favela when I first began fieldwork in 1998, but by the summer of 2009, my last sustained fieldwork visit, several families I knew had purchased private insurance plans for all or some members of the family, and the desire for private plans was expressed with increasing frequency.[3]

Self-Enhancement versus Self-Reproduction

While the explicit purpose of private medical insurance is to ensure entrance to the city's private hospitals and medical clinics, in Pirambu it also accomplishes several other feats. One of the more obvious is to introduce residents to a range of illness categories and medical consumables not previously imagined. A young woman I knew, Gisele, purchased private dental insurance through her job with a manufacturing plant and was delighted to see an extended brochure on orthodontics, including braces, which she was quickly persuaded she needed. In another case, a couple was worried about their daughter who wasn't eating much and was deemed too thin. The girl's father said he was reviewing the brochures of a private insurance plan he was considering purchasing when he learned about the disease anorexia nervosa. According to a brochure, the illness could be managed successfully through psychiatric medication and care, and he was eager to see if that would work for his daughter.

The process of medicalization, or introducing communities to new spectra of bodily ailments and therapeutic treatments, has been well documented by medical anthropologists (Lindenbaum and Lock 1993, Kleinman 1988, Scheper-Hughes 1992), and it has been operative in Pirambu for decades. The rapid expansion of clinical medicine during the twentieth century throughout Fortaleza ensured that Pirambu's residents relied less and less on their store of herbal knowledge, traditional healers, and the rare hospital visit for mortal illness and came instead to both desire and demand medical services and pharmaceuticals with which to treat an ever-expanding set of human ailments. The knowledge disseminated by private medical insurance plans can be understood as yet another space for the insertion of medical thinking and practice into residents' everyday lives.

Nancy Scheper-Hughes has argued of medicalization in the Northeastern city of Recife that health care practitioners including pharmacists were not part of a grand conspiratorial plot intended to coerce poor favela dwellers into a "dysfunctional dependency" but rather, recalling Gramsci's notion of hegemony, were part of an indirect and subtle transformation of everyday knowledge and bodily practice in which medical terminology and treatment became the obvious point of view (1992). And so, likewise, for the younger residents in the favela who disparaged public medical clinics and saved their hard-earned wages for private medical treatment and insurance, it was clear that they did so because they had come to share the views of those who sold the private insurance plans to which they aspired.

In contemporary Brazil, access to private medical insurance and care offers the young, urban poor an opportunity for self-enhancement that cannot be found through the consumption of public health care. Several studies have suggested that in Brazil certain medical procedures such as plastic surgery, caesarian sections, and the use of sex hormones can sometimes become a means of achieving social status for the urban poor (Béhague 2002, Edmonds 2007, Sanabria 2010). Let me return briefly to the two examples mentioned above, dental work and the treatment of anorexia nervosa, and describe how in these cases complying with particular medical regimes became a part of constituting oneself as an upwardly mobile citizen.

Gisele worked hard to obtain the job she held as a secretary at a local manufacturing plant. With her father's encouragement she was attending a two-year college at night and had saved enough money to purchase a private, employer-sponsored dental insurance plan. She told me she hoped to find a boyfriend from outside the favela and needed a "new mouth to do it." The public dental clinics that dotted the favela offered little more than tooth-pulling services, and paying out of pocket at a private clinic for the braces she wanted was out of the question. Dental insurance allowed her to pay for what she allowed was largely cosmetic work in installment plans matched to her monthly paychecks. What interested me most about Gisele's engagement of private insurance was the number of times she mentioned it to friends, extended family members, and co-workers. It appeared that even before her teeth were "made beautiful," possessing private insurance was for her a substantive marker of social mobility.

Private insurance and medical treatment also fit into the narrative of self-advancement in the case of the father whose daughter exhibited symptoms of anorexia nervosa as described in an insurance brochure. Vitor Silva, the girl's father, was the son of a moderately well-off postman in Pirambu. Vitor married at the relatively late age of thirty and worked as a delivery man for a company that sold computers in Fortaleza. He and his wife chose to have only two children so they could shower them with the resources more often associated with middle-class Brazil. When I met the couple in 2000, they lived in a spacious, light-filled apartment above Vitor's parents' home. In 2005 Vitor was promoted and transferred to Sobral, a sprawling, rapidly growing, hot city inland of Fortaleza.

During one of Vitor's return visits to Fortaleza he described to me his decision to move his family in terms of social mobility: "Our house is much bigger, my salary goes a lot further than it would here in Fortaleza, we might be able to send our girls to private school, and we were able to purchase private health insurance." This last advantage, he said, was especially important because his daughter had just been to a doctor in Sobral and was diagnosed with anorexia, a disease he wasn't aware of until reading about it in the brochure about private insurance plans. "I know that maybe you see it [anorexia] in some of the wealthier areas in Fortaleza, but here in Pirambu, no one's ever heard of it. There's no way it could have been treated by the doctors in the neighborhood. Now, with private medical care in Sobral we found the doctors and therapists we need." Though discouraged by the amount of money he was spending on medical care, Vitor was excited about the family's prospects for the future. "This is just a challenging period, but graças a Deus [thank God], we have the care we need, and with this promotion, in a few years we'll be able to return to Fortaleza to a better place."

In the two examples I've provided above, private health care was appealing to Gisele and Vitor not only because of the additional services it offered but specifically because in the favela private services also signify upward mobility, individual choice, and self-enhancement. The examples typify a younger generation of residents who do not aspire to improve the collective conditions of their community as their parents and grandparents did but rather to lift themselves and their immediate families out of the community altogether. These two cases also demonstrate how private health insurance and the services it buys offer another way to increase one's status in an increasingly competitive and unpredictable neoliberal economy (Edmonds 2007).

Os Miseráveis

The consumption of medical care by the younger generation in Pirambu did not always take place in the manner and according to the logic described above. The following case of a woman I knew named Josefa and her daughter Terezinha presents a startling contrast to the stories just related. Josefa was the wife of Neto and the daughter-in-law of Maria Clara. While Neto was quick-witted and ambitious, Josefa, his common-law wife, was widely presumed to be lazy, without ambition, and careless about domestic routines. Their union was assumed to be the outcome of an unplanned pregnancy, and the couple eventually had a total of four children. The couple fought often and publicly about conventional matters—money, liberty, and personal happiness. They lived around the corner from me during my first period of fieldwork, and their children were both wild and charming. I spent a considerable amount of time then taking comfort in and absorbing the routines of their household.

Josefa's self-proclaimed strategy when she ran out of patience or money (or both) for her children was to take as many of them as she could and leave them for as long as she could at her mother-in-law's house. Sooner or later Maria Clara would tire of caring for her grandchildren and having to worry about feeding four additional hungry mouths, and back the children would be sent to their mother, often with a sharp aside to Neto that he "had better start providing for his family and put a stop to his wife's begging." Here and there I heard stories that Josefa hadn't come from a *família boa* (good family), that she might be an orphan, and that they couldn't expect more when her own mother hadn't cared for her. And indeed Neto's extended family, though sometimes critical, did often seem to serve as a substitute for the many social relationships Josefa lacked.

As is probably apparent, Josefa bore almost no relationship to the women I have described earlier in this chapter: she didn't associate with them, she had children at a very young age (fifteen) even by the standards of the favela, she lacked any ambition to finish high school, let alone go on to college, and she seemed to have no plans or even imagination about what the future might hold. She also expressed very different views about health care than the other men and women I've described. In the spring of 1999, toward the end of my first period of fieldwork, Josefa's youngest daughter, Terezinha, was experiencing difficulty making bowel movements and crying each time she did so. Josefa took her for a checkup to the *posto infantil*, a small, public, pediatric clinic less than three blocks from where she lived, and then stayed with her daughter at the clinic for the next five days.

I hadn't seen Josefa for several days when her cousin asked if I wanted to come with her to the clinic for a visit. We walked to the clinic, which was in a clean, open-air building and somewhat crowded. We made our way to the large room where mother and daughter were staying, surrounded by four other infants who were also being tended by their mothers. Terezinha was happily chattering away with Josefa and looked by far the healthiest of the group.

She was diagnosed with ringworm, given medication, and then asked to remain with her mother at the clinic for observation. I wrote all of this in my field notes with an emphasis on what I considered most remarkable: "It's all for free!" As we entered the canteen where Josefa was eating her meals, she remarked that the food was especially good the past few days and that she thought she might not go home that day as we'd expected but would wait until the next afternoon. Josefa and Terezinha eventually went home a few days later with a bottle of ringworm medication and instructions on how to administer it. The problem seemed to have been largely cleared up, though Terezinha did end up back at the clinic a few weeks later for additional medication.

Talking with Josefa after she returned from the clinic, I was struck mostly by the things she didn't say: she didn't complain about the slowness of the service, the quality of the doctors, the ineptness of the staff, or the crowded, spartan rooms. Instead, she remarked that it was stressful to be home, where the daily worry of feeding her household had resumed. She didn't comment upon what I considered the most astonishing part of the clinic stay, that she hadn't paid a cent for any of it.

I present this narrative to showcase a distinction that was becoming more pronounced in the favela between younger residents who appeared to perceive and consume private medicine as though it were a form of self-enhancement and those who entered into publicly funded medical regimes partly as an opportunity to be recognized and attended to by the state. João Biehl has called this social practice "citizenship through patienthood" (2009); ironically, this is exactly the opposite of what the 1988 constitution intended; its language explicitly was meant to guarantee patienthood through citizenship. What I saw repeatedly was that for the urban poor struggling near or at the bottom of an already economically disadvantaged community, people whom more well-off residents of the favela refer to as "os miseráveis" (the miserable) or "pobrezinhos" (poor little ones), the mere ability to sustain oneself and one's family members day in and day out was so challenging that a venue like the calm lodging and meals at the public health clinic was perceived as an opportunity to attain socially recognized status as a person, in effect to constitute oneself as a citizen. And the more public health care became associated with residents like Josefa, the less interest residents like Gisele had in using it, thereby reproducing the very forms of social inequality that the constitution was intended to mitigate.

Narratives of Failure

An important question remained, however: What were the origins of the aspirations among the younger, more economically mobile residents? How, that is, did the aspirations of younger residents in Pirambu for privatized forms of medical care emerge from the broader political, social, and economic context in which they lived? The kinds of self-perceptions and aspirations I have attributed to the upwardly mobile, young residents reflect a form of subjectivity and a health ideology that have emerged in Brazil in the wake of the dictatorship and the subsequent shift to rights-based, democratic ideals on the one hand and neoliberal economic policies and practices on the other. In what follows I investigate how certain younger residents interpreted their social and economic circumstances in order to understand how for them public medical care slowly became associated with economic and moral failure in the favela. I then suggest that the programs begun under the auspices of the SUS such as Farmácia Viva and the Programa Saúde de Família (PSF, Family Health Program) encouraged a disciplined, individualized view of health care ironically best fulfilled by private rather than public health care services in Fortaleza.

Although the residents on whom I have focused were as a whole more economically secure than either their parents' generation or their less ambitious peers, the specter of failure was always close at hand. Among twelve young women whom I knew well in the favela and their extensive family networks, only one person held stable employment throughout the decade I conducted fieldwork. Everyone else experienced intermittent employment at a series of formal and more often informal labor sites. Thus even the younger, more advantaged residents had a constant sense that they were on the threshold of an event that could throw them and their families into economic chaos.

In this context, symbols of tangible success such as a high school diploma, training certificates, and stable employment were highly sought by this group of residents and interpreted as evidence of an eventual life *fora da favela* (outside of the favela), while intermittent employment, religious fanaticism, and being "uneducated" and "lazy" were disdained. Almost every one of the young women I knew had an example in her own family of someone she considered *muito mal educado* (very rude but also implying backward or badly behaved) and destined for failure.

Sofia, who was working as a masseuse, constantly criticized her older sister, Cláudia, and remarked on her inability to do anything positive with her life. Although Cláudia worked occasionally at a local beauty salon, Sofia complained that she spent most of her time "just hanging out." Sofia told me, "You know, she'll get up late and watch TV, talk with my aunts and uncles. It's like they do in the *interior*, just gossip all day long, and nothing ever happens."

For Sofia, her sister's laziness was implicitly connected to a lack of worldliness about life outside the favela. This was epitomized one day when I was visiting their family and Cláudia asked me when I was leaving to go back to America. I told her it would be another couple weeks yet, and she asked what bus I would take to get back home. "You see?" asked Sofia, exasperated, after her sister left. "She doesn't even know that you have to fly in an airplane to get to America!"

Even among friends judgments made about one another's work routines, personal lives, and spending habits were often linked to assessments of one's ability to achieve a life beyond the favela. One group of women I knew constantly fussed over a member of their circle, Olívia, who had worked at the same small gift shop for seven years. Although she eventually managed to graduate from high school, she consistently put off taking the *vestibular* exam that might have earned her entrance to the public university in Fortaleza, and she refused to take a series of easier tests that could have given her a place in one of the small, private colleges the other girls were attending. They made such remarks as "Olívia just lets herself be taken advantage of in this job" and "She doesn't really want to improve" and "As long as she can have fun on a Saturday night, she's happy." Typically these conversations would end with a statement like "What's going to happen in the future? She'll be fired eventually, and then what has she got?" and "She hasn't really made anything with her life, and she's going to be stuck in Pirambu forever."

The value this group of younger residents placed on creating lives for themselves and pursuing opportunities outside of the favela directly informed the opinions they held about public medical care. More than the quality of the services they received in public clinics, although they were critical of this as well, younger residents despised the comportment they were forced to assume in the process of obtaining such care. Waiting in long lines, sitting in the dimly lit, unair–conditioned halls of a tropical clinic, being treated anonymously once they finally did get in to see a doctor, and even the physical location of the public health clinics inside the favela were all reminders of living conditions they were actively trying to escape.

For these younger residents in the favela, rejecting public health care to the extent that they could and voicing complaints about it when they could not meant rejecting the passive, powerless, and unsophisticated ways of living that they associated with favela residents who were content to merely accept their lives as they were. In contrast, pursuing private medical care, even at great expense, provided tangible evidence of their success in operating outside of what they perceived as the favela's narrow borders. It meant knowing enough about how things worked in the city of Fortaleza to find a doctor to see, to find their way there, and to fit in with the other, presumably middle-class patients in the hushed waiting rooms when they got there.

In addition to spurring their desire for visible indications of financial success, the fear of failing, of being left behind in the favela, encouraged this group of younger residents to cultivate forms of self-discipline that would help them avoid economic and social marginalization. I have already mentioned some of the ways that self-discipline was exercised, such as identifying archetypal members of their families, like "the lazy sister," against which they could measure themselves. Other forms of discipline were learned at the colleges they attended and their places of employment. What I want to focus on next, however, is the forms of self-discipline encouraged by the public health care programs initiated by the SUS.

Health and the Cultivation of Self-Discipline

During my interviews with doctors and nurses who worked in Pirambu, they often stressed the type of health care residents in the favela received and how little the residents appreciated it. "Our aim," one of the young female doctors told me, "is to teach preventive care so that people don't end up at the big hospitals in the city. People here don't understand what a great opportunity this is. I can tell them, having a doctor visit you in your house—and to have that same doctor return to visit you a month later? That's amazing! I don't have health care that offers me this option—and I have a private health plan."

The program the doctor described here is the state *agentes de saúde* (health agents) program that sends nurse-directed health workers into communities throughout Fortaleza and the entire state of Ceará to carry out household visits once a month on a small number of priority health topics. The program was initiated in 1989 by the newly elected reformist governor Tasso Jereissati. His administration exercised taxation authority granted by the 1988 constitution to create this and several other basic health and social welfare programs. By 1997, the year before I started fieldwork, the program had nine hundred health agents working in Fortaleza and served 55 percent of the city's poorest residents (Svitone et al. 2000, 295). Identified by their bright-blue T-shirts that read "Agentes de Saúde" and blue jeans, health agents were a common sight in Pirambu. I spoke with them frequently during my first period of fieldwork in 1998–1999 to learn more about health conditions in the favela.

An individual urban health agent was typically responsible for visiting ten to fifteen homes per day, and each household was to be visited at least once a month. Agents carried with them knapsacks of supplies that included oral rehydration packets, soap, iodine, bandages, thermometers, and health records for each of the families they were to visit that day. As the agents told me repeatedly, their mandate was to provide health information, not to offer medical care. "Our goal," I was told by one of the health agents in 1998, "is really to help people understand what being healthy is. We just want them to know what they have to do to keep a clean house, to make sure their children are immunized. These are basic things they might not know otherwise."

One of the longest-running campaigns that I witnessed in the favela was designed to help residents prevent the spread of dengue fever, a sometimes life-threatening illness transmitted by mosquitoes. Because mosquitoes prefer to lay their eggs in open containers of stagnant water, the health agents' job was to inform households about how dengue fever spread and to encourage them not to leave open vessels of water around the house where mosquitoes might lay their eggs. During the health visits I observed either when I accompanied a health agent or was a visitor in a resident's house when a health agent paid a visit, the health agent typically asked if anyone in the house had had dengue and if they knew how the virus was transmitted. The more outgoing of the agents would then ask to look around the house to see if there were any open containers of water. They marked their family health record cards accordingly and went to the next household. These cards were then collected by a central program nurse who in turn reported the data to her supervisor at the state health department.

Although the program as a whole looked remarkably low-tech and informal, the data that health agents collected provided the city with in-depth statistics about the populations of the city's periphery and allowed officials to more accurately measure infant and child mortality rates, frequency of chronic illnesses, and living and education standards (Svitone et al. 2000). Thus programs like Agentes de Saúde helped to facilitate the SUS's broadest goal of bringing health care to all of Brazil's citizens by providing the data in granular and aggregate form through which favela residents were surveyed and their health habits analyzed. One of the health agents told me, "We've never had data about the individual families before. Now this allows us to institute population-based monitoring."

Although the health and physical well-being of populations has long been understood as a political objective in Ceará, collecting data on hundreds of thousands of individual families in peripheral neighborhoods helped public health officials to create, in concert with city politicians, targeted health and education programs for the poor. Foucault's description is instructive here: "The new noso-politics inscribes the specific question of the sickness of the poor within the general problem of the health of populations, and makes the shift from the narrow context of charitable aid to the more general form of a 'medical police,' imposing its constraints and dispensing its services" ("Politics of Health," 1984, 278).

The "medical police" of the twenty-first century were in this case the *agentes de saúde*, who spread like molasses through Pirambu, making their way from house to house, pulling out faded and often crumpled health records for families, on which they dutifully recorded pertinent information about the visit and proceeded to discuss that day's interventions. One of the first large-scale campaigns they undertook was to screen for illiteracy. In 1995 and 1996 *agentes de saúde* screened more than one million families in the state of Ceará to identify illiterate children ages eleven to seventeen and those of ages six to seventeen who were out of school. The names and addresses of these families were given to the local public schools, and within a year there was a 17 percent increase in elementary school attendance (Svitone et al. 2000). Besides earning Ceará national and international awards for the dramatic increase in the state's literacy rates, campaigns like this allowed health agents to define degrees of poverty, categories that were themselves put to use by the younger residents described in this chapter.

During my first extended fieldwork stay and on my return visits in the early 2000s, many *agente de saúde* interventions I observed focused on maternal and child health. I sometimes accompanied a health agent on a newborn visit to a family just after the baby was born, regardless of how many children the mother already had. The agent always asked about the health of the mother and the child, reminded the mother to breastfeed for as long as possible, and encouraged her to bring the baby to a clinic for monthly weight checkups. But in my subsequent returns to Pirambu, in 2005, 2007, and 2009, the instruction of health agents had shifted to include a set of self-care tips necessary to keep oneself and one's family healthy. "You can do this," the health agent told one bleary-eyed mother. "You just need to make more of a routine, to get yourself and your baby on a schedule. Be sure to write the clinic visits in your calendar. This should be part of the routine too." Mothers were reminded to visit their local health clinic on certain days of the week for a postnatal checkup and to be sure to take equally good care of themselves as they did of their babies.

The training of individuals to employ routines of self-care reminded me of conversations I'd had with doctors practicing in the favela who stressed the need to educate residents about how to be good consumers of health care. To ensure the efficient delivery of health care, doctors needed to normalize specific categories of medical care such as pre-natal and postnatal care and well-child visits, instruct residents when to avail themselves of such care, and train them to carry out certain health-seeking routines at home. Because the *agentes de saúde* visited residents in their homes, their purview spread to almost any household activity in need of discipline—from where to store water to how to care for one's baby to how to encourage literacy in children.

In a process similar to that described by anthropologist Sean Brotherton of Cuba (2012), these all-encompassing health campaigns led by the *agentes de saúde* effectively produced a new kind of medicalized subjectivity in Pirambu in which residents were encouraged to acquire a biomedical understanding of bodily health and physical well-being and were praised for complying with disciplined medical regimes. Other scholars have noted this attention to personal responsibility in the context of public health care in Brazil. Observing reproductive services in Bahia, Emilia Sanabria has noted, "Good patients are those who comply with medical protocols and display proficiency with regard to medical and institutional protocols" (2010, 282).

Chronic underfunding of the public health care system, however, meant that the experience of discipline and order being encouraged by the *agentes de saúde* was not what residents found if they dutifully made their way to local health clinics. A classic instance of this incongruity was a brochure I saw on the dirt floor of a woman's home that had been left behind by an *agent de saúde* who came to see her baby. The glossy brochure showed several mothers, one of whom was breast-feeding, in a spacious waiting room of what was presumably a public health clinic. "Veja seu SUS [See your SUS]," the brochure read, though the pictures were unlike any SUS clinic I'd seen in Fortaleza.

As I have tried to elaborate here, it was the younger, more aspirational residents of the favela who were particularly observant of and incensed by this discrepancy. While earlier generations organized communal social protests for better public care, the younger residents in the favela now channeled their significant frustrations into the consumption of individualized private health care, as the next narrative demonstrates.

Choosing Prenatal Care in the Favela

Vera Vaz was thirteen years old when I began fieldwork in Pirambu. I lived with her and her mother and grew to know her well during my extended stays in the neighborhood. Vera's mother, Isabella, made her *lambedores* (medicinal syrups made from plants) and herbal teas when Vera fell ill with the occasional flu or cold. I went with her to the nearest public clinic on one occasion when she had what turned out to be bronchitis, and I offered to help pay for the prescribed pharmaceuticals, which were out of stock at the clinic's hospital. Neither Isabella nor Vera commented on the quality of the health care they received, and in fact, the SUS was only a point of discussion when I brought up the topic.

As Vera grew up she made a close circle of girlfriends, most of whom came from slightly more comfortable backgrounds than her own and who had high expectations and aspirations for themselves and their peers. Her mother commented frequently on the quality of these women in overtly moral terms. "They're good people," she would say. "They treat Vera well and know how to get about in the world." She often voiced her hope that the girls' strong work ethic and self-discipline would rub off on Vera, though her desires for her daughter's future were not identical to the girls' own. Isabella envisioned her daughter living in a house to which she had legal title and working in a stable job with a fixed income, perhaps as a civil servant, while Vera's friends more often talked about moving out of the favela, owning cars, working in the private sector, and sending their children to private schools.

By 2009 Isabella had passed away and Vera was married and pregnant. On my last field visit I accompanied Vera to several prenatal appointments in Pirambu. Through SUS, all expectant mothers are entitled to ten prenatal visits throughout their pregnancies, including three ultrasounds, one each in their first, second, and third trimesters. They can go to any hospital to give birth as long as it has a maternity ward. Vera was twenty-six and, like other women her age, had been schooled repeatedly by the *agentes de saúde* and other health campaigns about the importance of prenatal care. And indeed, the visits seemed to be a growing point of pride for Vera and several of her friends who were pregnant at the same time. I remember standing in the recently tiled living room of Vera's grandmother's home with Vera and her cousin Fernanda,[4] who was also six months pregnant, while they compared notes about their pregnancies and discussed the doctors they had seen at prenatal care appointments.

They talked about the gender of each baby, a boy for Fernanda and a girl for Vera, and what color they wanted to paint the walls of the rooms where the babies would sleep; both thought they would choose yellow. And then Vera asked if Fernanda was going to the Posto de Saúde 4 Varas for her prenatal appointments. Fernanda nodded but said she had only gone twice so far because the wait was so long. Vera agreed, re-marking that she returned to the clinic three times for her latest visit before there was a doctor available to see her. "I'm thinking of asking Bruno's mother [her mother-in-law] if she could help us see a private gynecologist," she said. Fernanda looked envious and suggested, "Going to town would be best. You can be sure they do the ultrasound the right way. And in Fortaleza I can get the vitamins I need that they never stock at the clinics here in Pirambu." And then they returned to a discussion of names for the babies.

A few weeks later I went with Vera to her prenatal appointment. By then she had managed to persuade her mother-in-law to pay for an ul-trasound at a private clinic in Fortaleza, and Vera described her experi-ence to me: "It was beautiful, Jessica, completely beautiful. The build-ing was right in the center of the Aldeota, and you took an elevator six floors up. There was hardly anyone in the waiting room, and then I got my own room and we did the ultrasound very quickly. It was all over so quickly, I just got a prescription for vitamins and the nurse let me keep photos of the baby!" She proudly pulled these out and showed them to me and a few of the other women in the waiting room of the public clinic.

Finally we were called into a small office down a narrow corridor. A nurse weighed Vera and took her temperature, and then we sat and waited for the doctor. The dusty wall-unit air conditioner was barely functioning on this hot, humid morning, and we were both sweating by the time the doctor, a light-skinned, fashionably dressed young woman, arrived. She finished a conversation on her iPhone and turned her atten-tion to Vera and asked, "So how many months are you?" She asked sev-eral more questions and then admired the ultrasound pictures that Vera presented to her. "Beautiful, the baby is beautiful. Are you taking your vitamins?" the doctor asked. Vera told her that the clinic never had vita-mins in stock. "Well get your friend to buy them, then," the doctor said, laughing and motioning to me. "But it's true," she said, turning to me, and becoming more serious, "the public health care system sometimes doesn't have what the people need. That's why it's so important that the private system exists as well. This way, the residents can choose where to get care. If they don't find what they need here, they can go to a pri-vate clinic in town."

"But it's expensive," I commented.

"It's true, but they seem to find a way. What's important is that they have the option to do it," she said. Then the doctor resumed her discussion with Vera. She marked in her calendar the day Vera's baby was due and talked about the other appointments she would need to have before then, the vitamins she should expect to take, and the list of immunizations the baby would need once she was born.

Vera left the clinic with a long set of instructions and appointment dates for the remainder of her pregnancy and the start of her baby's life. Despite the doctor's attention, though, her comment to me as we parted for the day was that she would need to talk to her mother-in-law very seriously about helping to pay for her to go to a private medical clinic and perhaps for private medical insurance for the baby.

Conclusion: A Politics of Health

Health care reform in Northeastern Brazil, stimulated by the enactment of Brazil's 1988 constitution, integrated local, state, and national levels of care and preventive and curative medicine. The constitution's declaration of health as a universal right of citizens allowed the leaders of the state of Ceará to replace the old and ailing public health system with the Sistema Único de Saúde. At the time of its creation, the SUS reflected many of the leaders' aspirations for a system that expanded the right of access to health care to impoverished communities throughout the state and that encouraged new forms of citizenship, democracy, and civic participation. In the chapters of this book I have described residents' complex and even at times contradictory responses to these reforms and examined the local projects, strategies, and ambitions toward which health care reform has been directed in the community of Pirambu. I want to elaborate on several of my discoveries here.

Local Ambitions

The perception and practice of health care reform and its attendant expansion of civil rights depends upon one's generational and socioeconomic position in the intricate social landscape of the favela. In my fieldwork I observed that older residents of the favela relied on an extensive and, under the SUS, strengthened system of public health clinics for their medical care. While they activated long-standing networks of social reciprocity in order to access that care, the fact of free health care was most often attributed to their participation in and contributions to the city of Fortaleza's labor market or to their residence in a cosmopolitan capital city rather than in the state's rural hinterlands. Thus for older residents of the favela, health care rights are undermined both in practice by the social mediation needed to procure them and in theory by an ethos that understands those rights as belonging to particular categories of citizens, those who participated in the formal labor markets or reside in the capital rather than to all Brazilians by virtue of their national citizenship.

Younger residents of the favela, and particularly those who are economically and socially ascending, also pose a challenge to the conceptualization of health care as a right. In examining patterns of medical decision making in Pirambu, I observed that public and private forms of health care appeared to propose substantially different accounts of personal identity and morality for younger residents, who tended to embed observations about public health care within narratives of economic failure and anxieties over social status and often described the act of obtaining public care as humiliating. Encouraged both by a vast consumer culture and unwittingly by public health programs such as the *agentes de saúde* to conceptualize health in a highly medicalized, disciplined, and individualized manner, members of the younger generation in the favela sought to activate this vision of health through the consumption of private medical care.

The growing desire for private health care among younger residents in the favela also means that resources that are public and guaranteed by right of law are coming to be interpreted as being only for *os miseráveis*, the poorest of the favela residents. As public resources become stigmatized by their association with the socially and economically immobile poor, civil rights have been reinterpreted in some quarters of the favela as promoting access to private goods and services rather than as a guarantee of social equality. I find this phenomenon a predictable outcome of trying to expand civil rights within a neoliberal economic regime that understands citizenship itself as the ability to freely and successfully participate in the consumer market (Edmonds 2007, O'Dougherty 2002).

The poorest residents of the favela, about whom little has been said in this ethnography, incorporated the health care reforms into their lives in ways that are different again from the attitudes I have just outlined. If, following Aristotle, we submit that man is an animal born to life but whose existence with regard to the good life—to the life of a citizen—can only be achieved through full participation in social and political life (in Lord 1984), then there are residents of the favela for whom citizenship is an illusory prospect. I think of the people I knew whose energies were consumed by sustaining their daily lives, who had neither the time nor the aspiration to participate in local councils on health care actions or community-oriented projects, and who appeared to engage the services made available by the health care reforms with an attitude of exhaustion rather than entitlement.

But the state has consistently abandoned this particular population, and in its very confirmation of the constitutional right to health care for all Brazilian citizens, it perpetuates this abandonment by mistaking citizenship for a natural state of being and not, again following Aristotle, a status that is achieved through practical activity in the world. It is for these residents that the clinics of the Sistema Único de Saúde have become not just or even primarily spaces in which to be healed but places to find food, shelter, and respite from daily life in the favela. Patienthood in these instances has become a path toward citizenship, not a consequence of it.

The multilayered responses to health care reform in Pirambu reveal that the civil right to health has been evolving on top of a deeply entrenched public-private health care system whose invidious distinctions are themselves reproduced by the choices that residents of Pirambu make about medical care. In the area of health, it is not only the elites and middle classes who have withdrawn from the public sector but also an emerging and ascendant lower class for whom private health care has become an important marker of social status (Martins et al. 2008, Sanabria 2010). Although members of the older generation of the favela and the very poor continue to use public health resources, offering few opinions on the quality of those resources, they do so not out of pride or self-consciousness about what Brazilian citizenship confers. The public-private division in health care thus reproduces inequalities found in the society at large.

Old- and New-Fashioned Activism

Health care reform in Ceará has unfolded concurrently with a shift in the practice of civil rights and the forms of social movements in the favela. Over the course of my fieldwork in Pirambu I observed the waning of collective action and community organizations directed at gaining concessions from the state. In their place I saw the emergence of a consumer-oriented activism that was aimed at securing one's share of medical commodities and cultivating healthy behaviors and habits and that increasingly understood civil rights as the right to choose among the available tiers of health care services.

Following James Holston's trenchant analysis of democratic citizenship in the urban peripheries of São Paulo (2008), I have demonstrated that like the favela dwellers of São Paulo, residents of Pirambu began their activism in the realm of domestic life. Starting in the 1930s the earliest residents of Pirambu began to build their homes on the edge of the Atlantic just north of Fortaleza. In this process of autoconstruction they began to make demands on the city in the late 1930s and the 1940s for property rights, plumbing, health care, and security. Holston argues that the originality and force of this activism lay in its roots in the domestic sphere. My own research suggests that Pirambu residents' ideas of citizenship were shaped as well by their participation in forms of political engagement. As early as 1940 residents began embarking on protests, marches to city hall, and other forms of political opposition to gain concessions from the city of Fortaleza. In doing so they expressed their social needs and aspirations as a right of citizenship and, remarkably, were able to achieve a broad spectrum of services and legal recognition from the city of Fortaleza.

I have elaborated on the theme of collective action in Pirambu by demonstrating the continuing effectiveness of residents' dissent and political opposition in protecting and expanding their access to health care throughout much of the second half of the twentieth century. What was striking about the movements was the existence of a political consciousness that saw health care not as something that should be understood as a benefit of employment, as the policies of Vargas and the military regime suggested but as something that should be guaranteed by virtue of citizenship as eventually proposed in the SUS. Thus, I want to draw attention not just to the involvement of the poor in the expansion of specific medical services but also to how individuals become active subjects in the creation of health care ideologies (Brotherton 2012).

A measure of success of the decades-long tradition of political and civic activism in Pirambu and other urban peripheral communities throughout the country was the landmark constitution of 1988 that formally guaranteed the right to health care for all Brazilian citizens. In expanding the right to health care to all citizens, the constitution ushered in new definitions of democratic participation and community engagement. It stipulates that the health care system must be governed according to democratic criteria and include the participation of civil society in its decision-making processes such as establishing health councils at the federal, state, and municipal levels that would engage local residents in planning and supervising health care actions. The new forms of democratic participation were not always well received. City officials presented community participation in health councils as part of a broader project of deepening democracy in Fortaleza, while residents of Pirambu tended to see the same calls for participation as a shirking of responsibility on the part of the city that appears to be part and parcel of neoliberal forms of governance.

I also found that older residents were committed to their own forms of civic engagement. Many I knew were engaged in daily work that they explicitly defined as having helped to shape their neighborhoods and community; they cleaned neighborhood streets, organized food drives, held sewing circles and church events, and helped their friends and family members get by from day to day. But unlike participation in the city's health care councils, their activities were largely unrecognized and rarely remunerated by city officials. As opposed to earlier forms of social protest and expression, the current forms were unlikely to protect, let alone expand older residents' access to health care or other social services.

The shifts in the form of community participation have not gone unnoticed by those older residents I spoke with who were active in social movements of the 1970s and 1980s. I had many discussions with Airton Barreto, leader of Movimento Emaús Amor e Justiça (MEAJ), an organization that provides free legal aid in Pirambu and has a long history there. When I began my fieldwork in 1998 our first conversations largely centered on the possibilities that the Brazilian constitution and its recognition of social minorities might make it easier for residents of Pirambu to obtain civil justice. At that time, Airton stressed that the number of his clients had been steadily increasing in recent years and that they were becoming more, not less aware of their rights and how to use them.

My last conversation with him in 2009 took a different tone. We were discussing the increase of violence in the favela, endemic throughout Brazil and widely commented on by both younger and older residents. Cement walls lined with glittering shards of glass were becoming more common in Pirambu, and community leaders were worried about an increasing drug trade. Airton's wife wanted to move away from Pirambu, and they were discussing where else they might live in Fortaleza. Besides the violence, he told me, there was a decline in volunteers for his organization; the older residents expressed exasperation at finding time for meetings when they had their hands full with making ends meet. And he noted that fewer young people were interested in the movement. He was not optimistic about the future. "The younger generation is looking elsewhere now," he observed. "It's not about fitting in here or making a better life for themselves here. They don't think they need legal rights any more—just a lot of money!"

Airton's reflections on and disappointment in Pirambu's youth speak to the emergence of a trend in low-income communities around the city in which older forms of activism for social equity are being replaced by consumer concerns about the right to make choices in the marketplace. To explore this statement in more detail let me return to the scene of Vera's prenatal visit at the local clinic. Toward the end of that vignette, despite what had been, in my observation, a thorough examination by a seemingly professional and competent doctor, Vera expressed her keen desire to secure private medical care for herself and her baby. Throughout her visit, her disdain for the public health care system and idealization of and desire for private medical care was fluidly woven into her narrative and shared unselfconsciously with her doctor and me. I remember her commenting at length on the aesthetics of the private medical clinic she had visited. "It was so beautiful," she repeated to me several times, describing the interior of the building and her admiration of its hushed, upscale environment.

As health care becomes increasingly understood as a commodity in Pirambu, as something to aspire to and consume in the same way that finding the right room color or crib for a nursery might be, young residents like Vera focus their energies on procuring aesthetically and socially desirable forms of private medical care for themselves and their family members rather than organizing for the right of all residents in the favela to reliably access public health care. Like older residents' personal investments in their communities, consumerism is unlikely to safeguard or expand low-income residents' access to health care. To the contrary, I have argued in this book that it is precisely consumerism that has encouraged younger residents of Pirambu to make distinctions among themselves between the deserving, upwardly mobile, and aspirational poor and the undeserving, idle, and indifferent poor that ultimately serve to legitimize the two-tiered health care system in Fortaleza.

Doctors who worked in the favela often participated in this dynamic. In Vera's visit to the clinic, her doctor urged her to get prenatal vitamins from a pharmacy since the clinic often ran out of them. If she couldn't pay for them herself, the doctor reasoned, why not ask the rich American who was standing there with her to pay for them? Turning to me, the doctor noted that the public health care system sometimes didn't have what the people needed, and that was why it was important that the private system existed as well so people had options. The emphasis the doctor placed on opportunity and choice for low-income residents as opposed to broader issues of equity reinforces the perception that what was needed in Pirambu was not more political protests but better-educated, higher-income consumers of health care so they could effectively exercise their opportunities.

The decades-long tradition of social activism in Pirambu challenged the state to provide basic, life-supporting services, conceived not as commodities but as civil rights. The right to health care guaranteed by the 1988 constitution was conceived at least in part with the intention of meeting this challenge. But new forms of engagement in Pirambu, themselves shaped by Ceará's neoliberal economic environment, have shifted the practice of civil rights away from protests directed at achieving social equity and toward expanding individual freedom to exercise choice. These shifts in the form of social activism help to explain some of the contradictions in the history and current unfolding of health care reform in Ceará.

In Summary

Health care reform, understood as part of an ongoing process of social change, continues in Brazil, in the United States (amid great controversy at the time of this writing, as U.S. citizens debate the merits of the Affordable Care Act),[1] and in countries around the world as we struggle to define and defend who may confer stewardship over health resources and the health of populations. In this sense the principles behind health care reform reflect our most deeply held beliefs about what is necessary for human flourishing and our essential responsibilities to the most vulnerable among us. In the midst of this process people will continue to use the substance and detritus of reform toward their own local projects and ambitions. It is these particularities that anthropology excels in capturing and that can help us to understand how, for example, Brazilian health care reform based around the idea of human rights could both mitigate and perpetuate systems of social and economic inequality.

To attend to these complexities, I have chosen in this ethnography to focus primarily on health-seeking behavior. Like all forms of practice, health-seeking behavior, or medical decision making, grows out of the dialectic between existing medical discourses and institutional structures and the ways in which people engage with these structures. In seeking to present a historicized account of the two-tiered health care system in Pirambu, I have suggested that these arrangements should be seen as encompassing the objective constraints within which residents act as well as the concrete outcomes of their actions. When favela residents choose between public and privatized forms of medical care, they are making moves toward personal moral worth and social advancement while also reproducing a two-tiered health care system as a reified fact.

And so it was with Fátima, a patient of the public health system. I remember one of the final trips I took with her to the hospital in the city center. When I went to meet her early that morning, a quiet had descended on her small, dank house. Two of her children were still asleep in their nighttime hammocks, slung across the width of the living room, and three others had settled down and were watching cartoons on the small television set. There was an acrid smell of smoke in the room from a hastily built outdoor fire that warmed the morning coffee. Bits of rice and beans clung to the room's single, wooden table and spilled over onto the dirt floor. Fátima swept the remaining scraps of food off the table and turned to pull a worn handbag out from a pile of clothes in the corner. "Ready?" she asked me. And when I nodded she said, "Then, let's go." Waving to her children, she told them she'd be back in the afternoon.

We walked through the favela in the rising light and made our way down the dusty lanes and up to the broad avenue where the buses ran. We ran the final steps to catch our bus, and she climbed inside ahead of me and sat down neatly. Quiet the whole ride, which took nearly an hour, Fátima eventually climbed off the bus and walked toward the stark, white hospital building where she was to receive chemotherapy. Air conditioning and clean, white halls beckoned.

We took the elevator to the fifth floor, and there she stopped for a cup of water from the large coolers placed just outside the elevator doors on every floor. She walked down the long hospital corridor, toward her destination, stopping just once more before a basket of pastries, free that day for patients. Smiling back at me, she dropped several into her bag and then wrapped one for herself in a napkin and continued down the hall.

Notes

Introduction

1. The Society for Medical Anthropology's Policy Committee has compiled a useful compendium of essays on global health reform, available at http://medanthro.net/research/cagh/insurancestatements. In this regard it should be noted that Brazil was not the first country in Latin American to establish a universal health care system rooted in human rights. Cuba, for example, has predicated its health care system on an understanding of health care as a basic human right since 1959 (Brotherton 2012).

2. For a thorough assessment of Brazil's health care reforms see the World Health Organization report *Twenty Years of Health Care Reform* (Gragnolati, Lindelow, and Couttolenc 2013).

3. Throughout this book I use the terms "peripheral community," "low-income neighborhood," and "favela" to describe the community of Pirambu and others like it in Fortaleza. Younger and older residents of Pirambu most often used the term "favela" to describe and refer to their neighborhood, sometimes with a derogatory overtone but other times with affection or pride. Scholars have come to use terms like "low-income neighborhood," "peripheral community," "peripheries," and "popular community"—to list only a few—to draw attention to the social and political production of these spaces and to the mutual dependence and interrelationship of the city and its outlying areas. For an extended discussion of the relationship between the center and periphery see Holston 2008, 147–157. For a thorough discussion of the politics of using any one of the terms listed above, consult Janice Perlman 2010, 29–36.

Teresa Caldeira in a 2012 article has also drawn attention to the legal meaning of the word "favela" as a group of dwellings that are built on invaded land and thus whose residents do not own the rights to their homes (387). She carefully distinguishes between this form of housing and what she and James Holston have described as "autoconstructed" houses, in which the land is purchased and the buyers are entitled to home ownership (Caldeira 2012, Caldeira and Holston 1999, and Holston 1991, 2008). Pirambu was indeed originally a favela whose dwellings were built on invaded land in the 1930s. However, in a process I describe in chapter 1, much of this land has come to be owned by Pirambu's residents. The residents' use of the word "favela" and their lack of discomfort with it (an attitude I do not assume is generalizable to other cities in Brazil) has led me to employ the term as well. I have tried to use the word "favela" when I am speaking only about Pirambu or when referring to bibliographic sources or official institutions that use the term themselves (see, for example, notes 2 and 3 in chapter 1). I use terms such as "peripheral community" and "low-income community" when describing a broader set of neighborhoods in Fortaleza or Brazil and when intending to comment upon the historically produced nature of Pirambu's relationship to Fortaleza. But there are undoubtedly inconsistencies in this practice throughout.

4. The term "neoliberal" is used exhaustively in anthropological and social theory literature, often without a clear statement of its meaning. I use the term throughout this book to refer to a particular type of governance that emerged in the 1970s in the global North and South and became widespread in Fortaleza during the decade I was conducting fieldwork. David Harvey (2005) has described neoliberalism as the elevation of capitalism from a mode of production into an ethic, a set of political imperatives, and a cultural logic. Kingfisher and Maskovsky (2008) offer examples of policy shifts embraced in this form of governance that align with what I saw in Fortaleza, including the formation of public-private partnerships, privatization of public services, elimination or reduction of subsidies, and reform of urban fiscal policies to encourage gentrification and the securitization of elite residential and commercial areas.

5. The Portuguese term *o interior* (the interior) as used in Brazil is difficult to render in English. Equivalents like "the sticks" or "the boonies" or even "the country" do not convey its subtleties. The term broadly refers to the interior region of the Northeast, also known as the *sertão* (backlands), covered by a distinctive scrubby vegetation (*catinga*) adapted to the extreme climate. Many residents of Pirambu, however, use the term *o interior* to refer to literally any area in the state of Ceará that is not Fortaleza. And thus even a coastal town might be rendered as "o interior," as when an older woman I knew told me her mother still lived in the interior. When I asked where, she replied, "Camoeim," a medium-size coastal town north of Fortaleza. *O interior* can also be used to indicate a mental state. To say, for example, that a person has "the mentality of the interior" is to suggest that they lack the sophisticated ways of city dwellers. Although it is often used in a pejorative fashion, particularly by the younger generations, to mean naïve, backwards, small-minded, and coarse, it can also become a term of longing and nostalgia for times past. It is in all cases an explicit contrast with *a vida actualmente* (life here and now) in the city.

6. Paulina Salamo, Fortaleza's secretary of health, gave a radio interview at the Universidade Federal do Ceará on January 12, 2003, on Rádio Comunitária Dom Lino FM 104.9.

7. James Brooks, "Brazilian State Leads Way in Saving Children," *New York Times*, May 14, 1993.

8. For an extended discussion of the ethics of reciprocity and dependency

in the Northeast see Nancy Scheper-Hughes's magisterial 1992 ethnography *Death without Weeping: The Violence of Everyday Life in Brazil*, 98–127. Although Scheper-Hughes is describing social relationships as she saw them in the 1960s and again in the 1980s, her descriptions closely parallel an ethos I observed among older residents in Pirambu in the 1990s and 2000s.

9. The term "doxa" is originally from the Greek, meaning a common belief or popular opinion, and was in wide usage before being adopted by Bourdieu.

Chapter One

1. I use the word "favela" throughout this chapter, perhaps in too liberal a fashion, for reasons I discuss in note 3 of the introduction. I will briefly describe here some of the features of Pirambu that might not be typically associated with the term. "Favela" is most often translated as "shantytown" in English and loosely connotes provisional shacks hurriedly thrown together with improvised material such as plastic tarps, corrugated metal, and cardboard along dirt lanes on the outskirts of Brazil's major cities. Though this might have characterized the community's appearance at its inception in the 1930s, by the late 1990s there were few parts of Pirambu to which this description could be applied. When I arrived in 1998, most of Pirambu's residents lived in one- or two-room cinderblock homes densely layered along the dirt lanes and alleys that carved out the mile-or-so tract of land between the large boulevard Leste-Oeste and the Atlantic Ocean. There were also many paved roads in Pirambu and surrounding neighborhoods lined with multistory houses covered in elaborate tile and surrounded by decorative wrought-iron fences. Heterogeneity characterized the residences in Pirambu, as it did the residents themselves.

2. The total number of favelas in Fortaleza varies dramatically depending on how the borders of each favela are drawn and to what extent the favela itself is broken down into individual neighborhoods. Pirambu is formally composed of four neighborhoods: Cristo Redentor, Nossa Senhora das Graças, Tyrol, and Quatro Varas. However, I also heard people refer to other nearby communities as being part of Pirambu. According to a social service organization in Pirambu, there are more than three hundred favelas in all of Fortaleza if individual communities are counted as single favelas (Gonçalves da Costa 1995, 48).

3. The 2010 census of the Instituto Brasileiro de Geografia e Estatística (IBGE, Brazilian Institute of Geography and Statistics) lists Pirambu specifically as the seventh-largest favela in Brazil (Feitosa 2011).

4. Beginning in 1882, literacy—both reading and writing—became one of the criteria for voting in Brazil. This requirement was not eliminated until 1985 and produced disenfranchisement of the great majority of the population (Holston 2008). There were, however, instances in which the literacy requirement was overlooked. Historian Vítor Nunes Leal (2012 [1948]) has argued that in the Northeast, fraudulent means of garnering votes such as the creation of voters with false names and ignoring of the literacy requirement were standard practice during the 1930s and 1940s. Newspaper articles from Fortaleza docu-

menting politicians' interest in peripheral neighborhoods suggest that residents were likely encouraged to cast their votes despite widespread illiteracy in these areas.

5. The term *salário mínimo* is used throughout Brazil to evaluate the status of a particular job. One *salário mínimo* (about 300 reais, or $150, a month in 2005) was considered a low-paying job, but it was considerably better than jobs in the informal sector of the economy, most of which did not pay a stable wage at all. A job that paid three or four times the *salário mínimo* was what most of the residents I knew aspired to, while jobs that paid many times more than the minimum wage were simply unimaginable.

Chapter Two

1. The term *posto de saúde* (also called *centro de saúde, unidade de saúde,* and *posto médico* by residents of Pirambu) refers to the small health care clinics that are found in low-income communities in Fortaleza and throughout Brazil. These clinics vary in size but tend to be housed in modest structures; from them residents can obtain preventive health treatments from primary care doctors and the occasional dentist. The clinics serve a bounded and designated community and provide services to residents without charge. As I point out in this chapter, many of the clinics in Pirambu emerged before the implementation of the SUS, following a countrywide practice of fostering preventive medical care; thus their increased presence under the SUS was widely understood by residents as a continuation of the standard of care rather than an improvement upon it.

2. Despite the constitutional definition of health care as a responsibility of the state, 60 percent of all spending on health care in Brazil is still private— a higher share than in most other Latin American countries ("Health Care in Brazil: An Injection of Reality," *Economist,* June 30, 2011).

3. I use the term "welfare" here to refer to all programs, services, and policies aimed at the social and economic betterment of marginalized peoples (Ansell 2007). Different forms of welfare took on different ideological frameworks, which is part of what I intend to track in this chapter. That health care eventually became a distinct type of welfare is part of a broad ideological shift toward thinking about welfare in a compartmentalized and dismembered fashion (Foucault 1994).

4. For a detailed history of the Santa Casa de Misericórdias in Brazil see A. J. R. Russell-Wood's *Fidalgos and Philanthropists* (1968).

5. In "Politics of Health" Foucault describes the emergence of government attention to health as "one of the essential objectives of political power" in Europe (1984, 94). What is remarkable in the Brazilian case is that public health does not emerge as a policy focus until the early twentieth century.

6. As a point of comparison, note that the U.S. Congress established a National Board of Health in 1879, but it was terminated a short four years later, and public health remained thereafter largely a state and local responsibility (Starr 1982).

7. Despite the report's focus on the Northeastern region of Brazil, Ceará was actually not among the states surveyed for the report.

8. Again, I think it is useful to note that in the United States there were medical professionals whose views may have been roughly comparable to those of the *sanitaristas*, but they were rarely found in administrative positions, and political arguments about health were associated with marginalized leftist political groups. Health in the United States was and to a large extent still is understood primarily as a technical problem, not a political one.

9. Federal intervention in health policy was not always met with enthusiasm. Particularly in Brazil's southern states, where political leaders believed that health services should be centered in the states and municipalities, the extension of federal power was strongly opposed. Other voices of dissent came from the urban middle and upper classes, which argued that as long as Brazil's major cities were free from disease, attention should be shifted to more pressing matters of public policy.

10. The health care center movement began in America in the early part of the twentieth century but was losing political support by the 1920s just as it was being adopted in Brazil. For a detailed comparison of health care centers in Brazil and the United States see Luiz Castro Santos and Lina Faria's excellent article "Os primeiros centros de saúde nos Estados Unidos e no Brasil" (2002).

11. Many physicians in Brazil objected that an organization that provided coordinated medical services and related social services would threaten their private medical practices. American doctors actually voiced similar concerns, the difference being that they were already a formidable political lobbying force and helped to shut down the U.S. public health center movement in the early 1900s (Starr 1982, 194).

12. I use the terms "biomedical" and "biomedicine" throughout this book to describe that branch of medicine that Merriam-Webster's Online Dictionary defines as "medicine based on the application of the principles of the natural sciences and especially biology and biochemistry." Largely synonymous with "western medicine" or "conventional western medicine," the term "biomedicine" is used by anthropologists to draw attention to its foundational principles in biology rather than in convention or the west per se. Biomedicine became widespread and hegemonic in Fortaleza during the twentieth century through the adoption of public policies and health care practices partially traced in this chapter. Even in the late 1990s and the 2000s, however, the use of biomedicine was still regularly intermixed with herbal and folk remedies by many of Pirambu's residents.

13. The "Brazilian economic miracle" or "Brazilian Miracle" is the name given to the time of exceptional economic growth that occurred during the military dictatorship in Brazil, primarily under the ultraconservative leadership of Emílio Garrastazu Médici, who was in power from 1969 to 1973. The *abertura política* (political opening) is the name of the process of liberalization that the military dictatorship underwent in Brazil starting in 1974 and that concluded with the promulgation of the new Brazilian constitution in 1988 under a civilian government. For a detailed account of this period see Alfred Stepan's *Democratizing Brazil* (1989).

Chapter Three

1. Donna Goldstein's book *Laughter Out of Place: Race, Class, Violence, and Sexuality in a Rio Shantytown* (2003) is a model of close ethnographic attention to people's perceptions of more formal democratic processes. In her work she suggests that residents of a favela in Rio de Janeiro "conceive of the very possibility of citizenship through their immediate experience" (201). It is precisely the details of Pirambu's older residents' immediate experience that I have tried to elucidate in the latter part of this chapter and that I argue account for their indifferent reaction to the proposed health councils.

Chapter Four

1. Traditional medicine is composed of the health practices, approaches, and knowledge about plant-based medicines used to treat and prevent illnesses and maintain well-being. Residents of Pirambu and other low-income neighborhoods in Fortaleza used the terms *medicina popular* (folk medicine), *remédios caseiros* (home remedies), or simply *ervas* (herbs) when talking about the use of medicinal plants. I have translated all of these terms as "traditional medicine" throughout the book.

2. Phytotherapy is defined as the use of plant-based medicines to treat and prevent illness. The Portuguese term *fitoterapia* was used almost exclusively in publications about the Farmácia Viva program and by the scientists at the Universidade Federal do Ceará who began the program.

3. Translations are mine unless otherwise noted.

4. Federal universities in Brazil have historically played an important role in the health care sector (Escorel 1999). The national Ministry of Health operated through teaching hospitals at federal universities and tended to provide more sophisticated and higher-quality care than the hospitals funded by the Brazilian social security system could provide. The teaching hospitals generally received the more complex medical cases, which required costly interventions other public hospitals could not provide; by the end of the 1980s almost all university medical centers received federal funds (Kisil and Tancredi 1996, 390).

5. The issues at stake here could be seen as similar to those that many anthropologists and indigenous rights activists have discussed with regard to pharmaceutical companies using traditional knowledge in the search for profitable pharmaceutical drugs without compensation for the bearers of that knowledge (Greaves 1994; Greene 1998; Prance, Chadwick, and Marsh 1994). In the case of the WHO, however, traditional knowledge is not just a means to an end. Instead, traditional knowledge and resources are recast within a scientific paradigm and used as vehicles through which the categories associated with pharmaceutical drugs can be introduced. There are spectacular examples of the kind of exploitation associated with pharmaceutical companies—the development of drugs from the neem seed and the rosy periwinkle are cases in point. But I would argue that the literature on intellectual property rights tends to focus exclusively on these blatant cases of exploitation and thereby misses some of

the more subtle ways in which traditional knowledge and scientific knowledge are mediated.

6. For an account of the status of traditional medicine within the realm of medical anthropology see Shane Greene's analysis of the intermediated nature of biomedicine and traditional medicine in "The Shaman's Needle" (1998).

7. Although the pamphlet attributes these formal registration steps to the WHO, their origins can be traced to Germany and France, which were pioneers in the "officialization" of plant medicines (Gilbert et al. 1997, 340). Following the German convention, the creation of a monograph that describes a plant in terms of its toxicity, clinical use, and pharmacology has proven the increasingly accepted pattern for the officialization of medicinal plants. This procedure has been adopted by Brazilian scientists engaged in natural products research and was passed into formal law in Brazil in 1995 when the Brazilian Ministry of Health mandated that scientific evidence be brought to support the popular use of medicinal plants and that their efficacy and safety be established before they are used by public health clinics (339).

8. The recommendation that medicinal plants be registered with Embrapa, Brazil's oldest and best-known state-owned biotechnology firm, hints at the other kinds of social worlds where the plants could circulate. Although the explicit aim of Farmácia Viva is to fulfill social rather than economic ends, the link to Embrapa suggests that Fortaleza's municipal government may suspect that at some time in the future one of the plants will become economically valuable. If so, registering the plant with Empraba would be one way to claim intellectual property rights over the plant.

Chapter Five

1. I want to make clear that I am using the terms "older generation" and "younger generation" here to point to a set of shared experiences that residents themselves use in distinguishing between groups within the favela. "Older" and "younger" are thus loosely, not precisely correlated with biological age. See Julie Livingston's 2003 article for an excellent discussion of the importance of distinguishing between emic and etic age-related categories.

2. In an article exploring teachers' and doctors' informal medical practices in post-Soviet St. Petersburg, Anna-Maria Salmi notes (2003) that teachers often used their social networks rather than formal market mechanisms to procure medicine. In both St. Petersburg and Pirambu, personal favors were used to facilitate access to public resources. In Pirambu this process was understood as a form of reciprocity that had characterized social relationships in the favela for decades. See Salmi's article for a lengthier discussion of this process in St. Petersburg.

Chapter Six

1. There are some important exceptions to this trend. See, for example, Béhague 2002; Béhague, Gonçalves, and Dias da Costa 2002; Berman and Rose

1996; and Chernichovsky and Meesook 1986. What I hope to add to this literature is a more nuanced account of those low-income residents who are turning to private medical care and under what circumstances.

2. Throughout my fieldwork, residents and doctors working in Pirambu commented on the large number of children with asthma in the community. "All of the children have asthma in the favela," one of my neighbors told me. "It's because of the bad air we breathe here." Bad air and poverty were the most common explanations offered for what appeared to be high rates of asthma in Pirambu. The doctors I spoke with offered similar explanations, often concluding with statements like "Well, what did you expect? It's the favela, after all." The effect of poverty on the incidence of asthma in Brazil is an area of active research among public health scientists. Readers with a specialized interest in this topic might begin by consulting the 2008 article by Britto et al., which specifically addresses asthma among children who were patients of the SUS in the Northeast.

3. An article in *The Economist* of June 30, 2011, confirms that insurance companies have started marketing "low-cost plans to Brazilians who have recently left poverty." For example, some companies offer low-cost X-rays and blood tests to those who cannot afford full health insurance plans.

4. Fernanda is the same girl I discussed earlier who was prescribed growth hormones at age nine.

Conclusion

1. For an illuminating discussion of the Affordable Care Act and the ways that anthropologists can contribute to debates about the act and health care reform more generally, see the 2014 article by Horton et al.

References

Abreu Matos, Francisco. 1997. "Living Pharmacies." *Ciência e Cultura: Journal of the Brazilian Association for the Advancement of Science* 49, nos. 5/6 (September/December):409–412.

———. 1998. *Farmácias Vivas: Sistema de utilização de plantas medicinais projetado para pequenas comunidades.* Fortaleza: Edições UFC.

Akerele, Olayiwola. 1987. "The Best of Both Worlds: Bringing Traditional Medicine up to Date." *Social Science and Medicine* 24, no. 2:177–181.

Alencar, Irlys Barreira. 1992. *O reverso das vitrines: Conflitos urbanos e cultura política em construção.* Rio de Janeiro: Rio Fundo Editora.

Andaya, Elise. 2009. "The Gift of Health: Socialist Medical Practice and Shifting Material and Moral Economies in Post-Soviet Cuba." *Medical Anthropology Quarterly* 23, no. 4:357–374.

Ansell, Aaron. 2007. "Zero Hunger in the Backlands: Neoliberal Welfare and the Assault on Clientelism in Brazil." PhD diss., University of Chicago.

Araujo, Abrahão. 2012. "Access to Higher Education in Brazil with Reference to Prouni." *Higher Education Study* 2, no. 1 (March):32–37.

Arendt, Hannah. 2004 [1951]. *The Origins of Totalitarianism.* Rev. ed. New York: Schocken.

Aseby, Edgar J. 1997. "Andes Pharmaceuticals, Inc.: A New Model for Bio-Prospecting." In *Biodiversity, Biotechnology, and Sustainable Development in Health and Agriculture.* Washington, DC: Pan American Health Organization.

Barbosa, José B. 1994. *História da saúde pública do Ceará.* Fortaleza: Universidade Federal do Ceará.

Béhague, Dominique. 2002. "Beyond the Simple Economics of Cesarean Section Birthing: Class Contrast, Medicalisation, and Gender." *Culture, Medicine, and Psychiatry* 26, no. 4:473–507.

Béhague, Dominique, Helen Gonçalves, and J. Dias da Costa. 2002. "Making Medicine for the Poor: Primary Health Care Interpretations in Pelotas, Brazil." *Health Policy and Planning* 17, no. 2:131–143.

Berman, P., and L. Rose. 1996. "The Role of Private Providers in Maternal and Child Health and Family Planning Services in Developing Countries." *Health Policy and Planning* 11, no. 2:142–55.

Biehl, João. 2005. *Vita: Life in a Zone of Social Abandonment*. Berkeley: University of California Press.

———. 2007. "A Life between Psychiatric Drugs and Social Abandonment." In *Subjectivities: Ethnographic Investigations*. Berkeley: University of California Press, 397–422.

———. 2009. *Will to Live: AIDS Therapies and the Politics of Survival*. Princeton, NJ: Princeton University Press.

Biehl, João, Joseph J. Amon, Mariana P. Socal, and Adriana Petryna. 2012. "Between the Court and the Clinic: Lawsuits for Medicines and the Right to Health in Brazil." *Health and Human Rights: An International Journal* 14, no. 1:1–17.

Biehl, João, and Adriana Petryna. 2011. "Bodies of Rights and Therapeutic Markets." *Social Research* 78, no. 2:359–394.

Bógus, Cláudia Maria. 1998. *Participacão popular em saúde: Formação política e desenvolvimento*. São Paulo: Anna Blume.

Bourdieu, Pierre. 1977. *Outline of a Theory of Practice*. Cambridge, England: Cambridge University Press.

Braga, Elza Maria Franco. 1991. *A política da escassez: Lutas urbanas e programas sociais governamentais*. Fortaleza: Universidade Federal do Ceará, Fundação Democrática Rocha.

Brito, Danielle de. 1996. "O movimento popular do Pirambu e a crise contemporânea: Uma análise da grande entidade." Bachelor of arts thesis, Universidade Estadual do Ceará.

Britto, Carlos Amorim de, Emilses Freire, Patrícia Bezerra, Rita Moraes de Brito, and Joakim Regos. 2008. "Baixa renda como fator de proteção contra asma em crianças e adolescentes usuários do Sistema Único de Saúde." *Jornal Brasileiro de Pneumologia* 34, no. 5:251–255.

Brodwin, Paul. 1996. *Medicine and Morality in Haiti: The Contest for Healing Power*. Cambridge, England: Cambridge University Press.

Brooks, Reuben Howard. 1972. "Flight from Disaster: Drought Perception as a Force in Migration from Ceará, Brazil." PhD diss., University of Colorado, Boulder.

Brooks, Sarah. 2008. *Social Protection and the Market in Latin America: The Transformation of Social Security Institutions*. Cambridge, England: Cambridge University Press.

Brotherton, Sean P. 2012. *Revolutionary Medicine: Health and the Body in Post-Soviet Cuba*. Durham, NC: Duke University Press.

Bryant, John. 1980. "WHO's Program of Health for All by the Year 2000: A Macrosystem for Health Policy Making—A Challenge to Social Science Research." *Social Science and Medicine* 14A, no. 5:381–386.

Burchell, Graham. 1996. "Liberal Government and Techniques of the Self." In *Foucault and Political Reason. Liberalism, Neo-Liberalism, and Rationalities of Government*, ed. Andrew Barry, Thomas Osborne, and Nikolas Rose, 19–36. Chicago: University of Chicago Press.

Caldeira, Teresa. 2006. "'I Came to Sabotage Your Reasoning!': Violence and

Resignifications of Justice in Brazil." In *Law and Disorder in the Postcolony*, ed. Jean Comaroff and John Comaroff, 102–149. Chicago: University of Chicago.

———. 2012. "Imprinting and Moving Around: New Visibilities and Configurations of Public Space in São Paulo." *Public Culture* 24, no. 2:385–419.

Caldeira, Teresa, and James Holston. 1999. "Democracy and Violence in Brazil." *Comparative Studies in Society and History* 41, no. 4 (October):691–729.

———. 2005. "State and Urban Space in Brazil: From Modernist Planning to Democratic Interventions." In *Global Assemblages: Technology, Politics, and Ethics as Anthropological Problems*, ed. Aiwha Ong and Stephan J. Collier, 393–416. Oxford, England: Blackwell.

Castro Santos, Luiz. 1987. "Power, Ideology, and Public Health in Brazil 1889–1930." PhD diss., Harvard University.

Castro Santos, Luiz, and Lina Faria. 2002. "Os primeiros centros de saúde nos Estados Unidos e no Brasil: Um estudo comparativo." *Teoria e Pesquisa* 40 (January/July):137–184.

Ceará, Governo do Estado do. 1967. *As migracões para Fortaleza*. Fortaleza: Departamento de Imprensa Oficial da Secretaria de Administração, Ceará.

———, Secretaria de Saúde. 1995. "Programa estadual de fitoterapia." Fortaleza.

Chernichovsky, D., and O. A. Meesook. 1986. "Utilization of Health Services in Indonesia." *Social Science and Medicine* 23, no. 6:611–620.

Coelho, Vera Schattan. 2007. "Brazilian Health Councils: Including the Excluded?" In *Spaces for Change? The Politics of Citizen Participation in New Democratic Arenas*, ed. Andrea Cornwall and Vera Schattan Coelho, 33–54. London: Zed Books.

———. 2013. "What Did We Learn about Citizen Involvement in the Health Policy Process: Lessons from Brazil." *Journal of Political Deliberation* 9, no. 1:1–17.

Collier, Jane. 2001. "Durkheim Revisited: Human Rights as the Moral Discourse for the Postcolonial, Post–Cold War World." In *Human Rights: Concepts, Contests, and Contingencies*, ed. Austin Sarat and Thomas R. Kearns, 63–88. Ann Arbor: University of Michigan Press.

Comaroff, Jean. 1994. "The Diseased Heart of Africa: Medicine, Colonialism, and the Black Body." In *Knowledge, Power, and Practice: The Anthropology of Medicine and Everyday Life*, ed. Shirley Lindenbaum and Margaret Lock, 305–329. Berkeley: University of California Press.

Cornwall, Andrea. 2007. "Democratizing the Governance of Health Services: The Case of Cabo de Santo Agostino, Brazil." In *Spaces for Change? The Politics of Citizen Participation in New Democratic Arenas*, ed. Andrea Cornwall and Vera Schattan Coelho, 155–179. London: Zed Books.

———. 2008. "Deliberating Democracy: Scenes from a Brazilian Municipal Health Council." *Politics and Society* 36:508–531.

Cornwall, Andrea, Silvia Cordeiro, and Nelson Giordano Delgado. 2006. "Rights to Health and Struggles for Accountability in a Brazilian Municipal Health Council." In *Rights, Resources, and the Politics of Accountability*, ed. Peter Newell and Joanna Wheeler, 144–161. London: Zed Books.

Crespo, Noe, Guadelupe Ayala, Christopher Vercammen-Grandjean, Donald

Lymen, and John Elder. 2011. "Socio-demographic Disparities of Childhood Asthma." *Journal of Child Health Care* 15, no. 4:358–369.

Dagnino, Evelina. 2005. "'We All Have Rights, But . . .': Contesting Concepts of Citizenship in Brazil." In *Inclusive Citizenship: Meanings and Expressions,* ed. Naila Kabeer, 149–163. London: Zed Books.

———. 2007. "Dimensions of Citizenship in Contemporary Brazil." *Fordham Law Review* 75, no. 5:2469–2482.

Edmonds, Alexander. 2004. "Learning to Love Yourself: Esthetics, Health, and Therapeutics in Brazilian Plastic Surgery." *Ethnos* 74, no. 4 (December): 465–489.

———. 2007. "The Poor Have the Right to Be Beautiful: Cosmetic Surgery in Neoliberal Brazil." *Journal of the Royal Anthropological Institute* 13, no. 2:363–381.

———. 2010. *Pretty Modern: Beauty, Sex, and Plastic Surgery in Brazil.* Durham, NC: Duke University Press.

Escobar, Arturo. 1995. *Encountering Development: The Making and Unmaking of the Third World.* Princeton, NJ: Princeton University Press.

Escorel, Sarah. 1999. *Reviravolta na saúde: Origem e articulação do movimento sanitário.* Rio de Janeiro: Editora Fiocruz.

Farias, Aírton de. 1997. *História do Ceará: Dos índios à geração cambeba.* Fortaleza: Tropical.

Farmer, Paul. 2003. *Pathologies of Power: Health, Human Rights, and the New War on the Poor.* Berkeley: University of California Press.

Farquhar, Judith. 1994. *Knowing Practice: The Clinical Encounter of Chinese Medicine.* Boulder, CO: Westview Press.

Feitosa, Angélica. 2011. "Pirambu: A maior favela do Ceará e a 7ª maior do Brasil." *O Povo Online,* December 22.

Ferguson, James. 1990. *The Anti-Politics Machine: "Development," Depoliticization, and Bureaucratic Power in Lesotho.* Cambridge, England: Cambridge University Press.

Ferraz, Octávio Luiz Motta. 2009. "The Right to Health in the Courts of Brazil: Worsening Health Inequities?" *Health and Human Rights: An International Journal* 11, no. 2:33–45.

———. 2011. "Health Inequalities, Rights, and Courts: The Social Impact of the 'Judicialization of Health' in Brazil." In *Litigating Health Rights: Can Courts Bring More Justice to Health Systems?,* ed. Alicia Ely Yamin and Siri Gloppen, 76–102. Cambridge: Harvard University Press.

Fleury, Sonia. 1997. *Democracia e saúde: A luta do CEBES.* São Paulo: Lemos Editorial.

Forment, Carlos A. 2003. *Civic Selfhood and Public Life in Mexico and Peru.* Vol. 1 of *Democracy in Latin America.* Chicago: University of Chicago Press.

Fortaleza, Prefeitura Municipal de. 1998. *Registro de medicamentos fitoterápicos.* Pamphlet.

———. 1999. "Estruturação e organização da fitoterapia na saúde pública do município de Fortaleza."

Fortaleza, Prefeitura Municipal de, Programa Farmácias Vivas. 1998. "Guia fitoterápico."

Fortaleza, Prefeitura Municipal de, Secretaria de Desenvolvimento Social. 1996. "Planta medicinal: Saúde para quem usa corretamente."

———. 1997a. "Quadrinhos da Saúde no. 1: Farmácias Vivas."

———. 1997b. "Quadrinhos da Saúde no. 3: Uso racional de medicamentos e fitoterápicos."

Fortaleza, Prefeitura Municipal de, and Sociedade Alemã de Cooperação Técnica. 1992. *Plano de desenvolvimento comunitário integrado.*

Foucault, Michel. 1984. *The Foucault Reader.* Ed. Paul Rabinow. New York: Pantheon Books.

———. 1994. *Power.* Ed. James D. Faubion. New York: New Press.

Freyre, Giberto. 1987 [1933]. *The Masters and the Slaves: A Study in the Development of Brazilian Civilization.* Trans. Samuel Putman. Berkeley: University of California Press.

Galvanezzi C. 2004. *Representação popular nos conselhos de saúde.* São Paulo: Fundação de Amparo à Pesquisa do Estado de São Paulo (FAPESP).

Gilbert, Benjamin, Jose L. P. Ferreira, M. Beatriz Almeida, Eliane S. Carvalho, Vera Cascon, and Leandro M. Rocha. 1997. "The Official Use of Medicinal Plants in Public Health." *Ciência e Cultura: Journal of the Brazilian Association for the Advancement of Science* 49, nos. 5/6 (September/December):339–344.

Goldstein, Donna M. 2003. *Laughter Out of Place: Race, Class, Violence, and Sexuality in a Rio Shantytown.* Berkeley: University of California Press.

Gonçalves da Costa, Maria. 1995. *Historiando o Pirambu.* Fortaleza: Seriartes Edições.

Gragnolati, Michele, Magnus Lindelow, and Bernard Couttolenc. 2013. *Twenty Years of Health System Reform in Brazil.* July. Geneva: World Health Organization.

Gramsci, Antonio. 1971. *Selections from the Prison Notebooks.* New York: International.

Greaves, Tom. 1994. *Intellectual Property Rights for Indigenous Peoples: A Source Book.* Society for Applied Anthropology.

Greene, Shane. 1998. "The Shaman's Needle: Development, Shamanic Agency, and Intermedicality in Aguaruna Lands, Peru." *American Ethnologist* 25, no. 4:634–658.

Harvey, David. 2005. *A Brief History of Neoliberalism.* Oxford, England: Oxford University Press.

Hayden, Cori. 2003. *When Nature Goes Public: The Making and Unmaking of Bioprospecting in Mexico.* Princeton, NJ: Princeton University Press.

Hirschfield, Katherine. 2008. *Health, Politics, and Revolution in Cuba Since 1898.* New Brunswick, NJ: Transaction.

Holmes, Seth. 2013. *Fresh Fruit, Broken Bodies: Migrant Farmworkers in the United States.* Berkeley: University of California Press.

Holston, James. 1991. "Autoconstruction in Working-Class Brazil." *Cultural Anthropology* 6, no. 4:447–465.

———. 2008. *Insurgent Citizenship: Disjunctions of Democracy and Modernity in Brazil.* Princeton, NJ: Princeton University Press.

Horton, Sarah, Cesar Abadia, Jessica Muligan, and Jennifer Jo Thompson. 2014. "Critical Anthropology of Global Health 'Takes a Stand' Statement:

A Critical Medical Anthropological Approach to the U.S.'s Affordable Care Act." *Medical Anthropology Quarterly* 28, no. 1:1–22.

Jacobi, Pedro. 2000. *Políticas sociais e a ampliação de cidadania.* São Paulo: Editoria da FGV.

Kingfisher, Catherine, and Jeffery Maskovsky. 2008. "Introduction: The Limits of Neoliberalism." *Critique of Anthropology* 28, no. 2:115–126.

Kisil, Marcos, and Francisco Tancredi. 1996. "The Brazilian Health Care Delivery System: A Challenge for the Future." In *At the Edge of Development: Health Crises in a Transitional Society,* ed. Richard L. Guerrant, M. Auxiliadora De Souza, and Marilyn K. Nations, 379–399. Durham, NC: Carolina Academic Press.

Kleinman, Arthur. 1988. *The Illness Narratives: Suffering, Healing, and the Human Condition.* New York: Basic Books.

Leal, Vítor Nunes. 2012 [1948]. *Coronelismo, enxada e voto: O municiípio e o regime representativo no Brasil.* 4th edition. São Paulo: Companhia das Letras.

Levine, Robert. 1981. "Urban Workers under the Brazilian Republic, 1889–1937." Occasional Papers no. 36. Glasgow, Scotland: Institute of Latin American Studies, University of Glascow.

Lindenbaum, Shirley, and Margaret Lock, eds. 1993. *Knowledge, Power, and Practice: The Anthropology of Medicine and Everyday Life.* Berkeley: University of California Press.

Lins, Luizianne. 2005. "Fortaleza: The Campaign That Relied on the Militants." Interview in *Democracia Socialista* 8 (November–December 2004); republished in English translation in *International Viewpoint* 363 (January), http://internationalviewpoint.org/spip.php?article238.

Livingston, Julie. 2003. "Pregnant Children and Half-Dead Adults: Modern Living and the Quickening Life Cycle in Botswana." *Bulletin of the History of Medicine* 77, no. 1 (Spring):133–162.

Lord, Carnes, trans. 1984. Aristotle, *The Politics.* Chicago: University of Chicago Press.

Magalhães, M. 1980. "A política de saúde pública no Brasil nos últimos 50 anos." In *Câmara dos Deputados, I Simpósio sobre Política Nacional de Saúde,* vol. 1: *Conferências.* Brasília, Coordenação de Publicações, Governo Federal do Brasil.

Martins, Poliana Cardosa, Rosangela Cotta, Fábio Mendes, Sylvia Franceschini, Silvia Priore, and Glauce Dias. 2008. "Conselhos de saúde e a participação social no Brasil: Matizes da utopia." *Physis Revista de Saúde Coletiva* 18, no. 1:105–121.

Marx, Karl. 1977. *Capital.* Vol. 1. New York: Vintage.

———. 1978. *The Marx-Engles Reader.* Ed. Robert C. Tucker. 2nd ed. New York: Norton.

Mechanic, David. 1999. "Issues in Promoting Health." *Social Science and Medicine* 48, no. 6:711–718.

McCullum, Cecilia. 2005. "Explaining Caesarean Section in Salvador da Bahia, Brazil." *Sociology of Health and Illness* 2 (March 27):215–242.

Mock, Kathryn L. 1997. "The Municipalization of Women's Reproductive Health Services in Ceará, Brazil." Master's thesis, University of Texas, Austin.

Morgan, Lynn. 1993. *Community Participation in Health: The Politics of Primary Care in Costa Rica*. Cambridge, England: Cambridge University Press.

Mors, Walter B. 1997. "Looking at the Origins." *Ciência e Cultura: Journal of the Brazilian Association for the Advancement of Science* 49, nos. 5/6 (September/December):310–315.

Mota, Maria Vaudelice. 1997. "Evolução organizacional da Secretaria da Saúde do Município de Fortaleza." Master's thesis, Universidade Federal do Ceará.

Moyn, Samuel. 2010. *The Last Utopia: Human Rights in History*. Cambridge: Harvard University Press.

Muehlebach, Andrea. 2011. "On Affective Labor in Post-Fordist Italy." *Cultural Anthropology* 26, no. 1:59–82.

Nobre, Maria do Socorro Silva. 1978. *História da medicina no Ceará (período colonial)*. Fortaleza: Secretaria de Cultura, Desporte e Promoção Social, Governo do Ceará.

O'Dougherty, Maureen. 2002. *Consumption Intensified: The Politics of Middle-Class Daily Life in Brazil*. Durham, NC: Duke University Press.

Paim, J., C. Travassos, C. Ameida, L. Bahia, and J. Macinko. 2011. "The Brazilian Health System: History, Advances, and Challenges." *Lancet* 377, no. 9779 (May 21):1778–1797.

Paley, Julia. 2001. *Marketing Democracy: Power and Social Movements in Post-Dictatorship Chile*. Berkeley: University of California Press.

Perlman, Janice. 1976. *The Myth of Marginality: Urban Poverty and Politics in Rio de Janeiro*. Berkeley: University of California Press.

———. 2010. *Favela: Four Decades of Living on the Edge in Rio de Janeiro*. Oxford, England: Oxford University Press.

Prance, Ghillean, Derek Chadwick, and Joan Marsh. 1994. *Ethnobotany and the Search for New Drugs*. New York: John Wiley and Sons.

Preis, Ann-Belinda. 1996. "Human Rights as Cultural Practice: An Anthropological Critique." *Human Rights Quarterly* 18, no. 2:286–315.

Rose, Nikolas. 1999. *Powers of Freedom: Reframing Political Thought*. Cambridge, England: Cambridge University Press.

———. 2007. *The Politics of Life Itself: Biomedicine, Power, and Subjectivity in the Twenty-First Century*. Princeton, NJ: Princeton University Press.

Russell-Wood, A. J. R. 1968. *Fidalgos and Philanthropists: The Santa Casa da Misericórdia of Bahia, 1550–1755*. Berkeley: University of California Press.

Salmi, Anna-Maria. 2003. "Health in Exchange: Teachers, Doctors, and the Strength of Informal Practices in Russia." *Culture, Medicine, and Psychiatry* 27:109–130.

Sanabria, Emilia. 2010. "From Sub- to Super-Citizenship: Sex Hormones and the Body Politic in Brazil." *Ethnos* 75 (December):4.

Santiago, A. P. 1996. "Histórico do Pirambu, 1996." Photocopy. Special Collections, Centro Popular de Pesquisa Documentação e Comunicação, Pirambu, Fortaleza.

Scheper-Hughes, Nancy. 1992. *Death without Weeping: The Violence of Everyday Life in Brazil*. Berkeley: University of California Press.

———. 2006. "Death Squads and Democracy in Northeast Brazil." In *Law and Disorder in the Postcolony*, ed. Jean Comaroff and John Comaroff, 150–187. Chicago: University of Chicago.

Silva, Geraldo Walmir. 1999. *Memória viva do Pirambu: O velho Pirambu de muletas nas mãos*. Fortaleza: Seriartes Edições.

Starr, Paul. 1982. *The Social Transformation of American Medicine: The Rise of a Sovereign Profession and the Making of a Vast Industry*. New York: Basic Books.

Stepan, Alfred C. 1989. *Democratizing Brazil: Problems of Transition and Consolidation*. Oxford, England: Oxford University Press.

Stone, L. 1986. "Primary Health Care for Whom? Village Perspectives from Nepal." *Social Science and Medicine* 22:293–302.

Stralen, Cornelis J. 1996. "The Struggle over a National Health Care System: The Movimento Sanitario and Health Policy-Making in Brazil: 1960–1990." PhD diss., Universiteit van Utrecht.

Svitone, Ennio Cufino, Richard Garfield, Maria Ines Vasconcelos, and Villane Araujo Craveiro. 2000. "Primary Health Care Lessons from the Northeast of Brazil: The Agentes de Saúde Program." *Revista Panam Salud Pública/Pan Am Journal of Public Health* 7, no. 5:293–301.

Teixeira, Sonia F. 1989. *Reforma sanitária: Em busca de uma teoria*. São Paulo: Abrasco/Cortez.

Ugalde A. 1985. "Ideological Dimensions of Community Participation in Latin American Health Programs." *Social Science and Medicine* 21, no. 1:41–53.

Van der Geest, Sjaak, Johan D. Speckman, and Pieter H. Streefland. 1990. "Primary Health Care in a Multi-Level Perspective: Towards a Research Agenda." *Social Science and Medicine* 30, no. 9:1025–1034.

Victora, Cesar G., Estela Aquino, Maria Leal, Carlos Monteiro, Fernando Barros, and Celia Szwarcwald. 2011. "Maternal and Child Health in Brazil: Progress and Challenges." *Lancet* 377, no. 9780:1863–1876.

Wheeler, Joanna. 2005. "Rights without Citizenship? Participation, Family, and Community in Rio de Janeiro." In *Inclusive Citizenship: Meanings and Expressions*, ed. Naila Kabeer, 99–113. London: Zed Books.

Win, Peter. 1989. *Weavers of Revolution: The Yarur Workers and Chile's Road to Socialism*. Oxford, England: Oxford University Press.

Index

CPSIA information can be obtained
at www.ICGtesting.com
Printed in the USA
BVHW040821141022
649429BV00001B/17

9 781477 311318